My Wonderful Life with Diabetes

An Inspiring and Empowering Story
of Living Healthy, Living Active,
and Living Well with Diabetes

By Rick Mystrom

Published by Tadfield Publishing LLC
in cooperation with Publishing Consultants

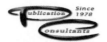

PO Box 221974 Anchorage, Alaska 99522-1974
books@publicationconsultants.com—www.publicationconsultants.com

ISBN 978-1-59433-393-4

eBook ISBN Number: 978-1-59433-394-1

Library of Congress Catalog Card Number: 2013942965

Copyright 2013 Rick Mystrom

—First Edition—

Printed In China.

Dedication

To my family who, without ever
knowing, gave me the reason and
motivation every day to stay healthy.

To order copies of this book or the author's upcoming book,

The New Diabetic Lifestyle,

go to RickMystrom.com

Table of Contents

Information Sources

The primary source of information in this book is my own memory.

To expand on my memory and verify details, I relied on my wife, Mary, and my three children, Nick, Rich and Jen. My friends, Asa Morton, Steve Kinney, Derek Gable, Rick Nerland, and Bill McKay were indispensible in sharpening details that have faded over the years.

I also drew from notebooks of thoughts and inspirational notes I wrote during my early days with diabetes as well as more than 45 years of calendars and meeting notes I have kept.

To add substance and specifics to my memory, I relied heavily on newspaper articles primarily from the *Anchorage Daily News*, *The Anchorage Times*, *The New York Times*, and the *Salt Lake City Deseret News*.

Finally my Olympic speeches and my boxes of Anchorage's Olympic bid records provided many direct quotes and references. Many of these records have been donated to the University of Alaska, Anchorage library and have been preserved in the UAA archives.

Foreword

Anchorage's bid for the Winter Olympics created among a diverse group of Alaskans friendships that have stood the test of time. When I first officially, but briefly, met Rick, I would never in my wildest dreams have predicted that more than 30 years later we would be in the middle of Africa together when his insulin pump failed with no replacement at hand. As a physician and friend, I got him some back-up syringes while he used a satellite phone to try to get a replacement pump. Amazingly, he got one.

Rick and Mary, and my wife, Ruth, and I moved to Anchorage in the same year. But it was not until Mystrom Advertising had been in existence for several years that I started to hear references to him as an emerging public figure of some stature.

This was an understatement! Looking at his involvement in the dramatic transformations of Anchorage and Alaska in the '80s and '90s, one begins to understand his inspirations, motivations, style, and philosophy of service.

To really know what makes Rick tick, you must understand a bit about diabetes and his trials and errors over the years in not only surviving the diagnosis, but actually thriving because of it. His diabetes weaves in and out of stories about both his public and private life. He says on balance it has been a positive influence and, in fact, he probably would not be as healthy as he is today if he had not had diabetes. His diagnosis of insulin-dependent diabetes at age 20 was a clarion call for him to understand his disease and take charge of his health. He wins the Olympic gold medal in both of these categories.

As Rick's story unfolds, I was struck by several recurring themes: management and attitude.

Effectively managing tight control of his diabetes is a partnership deal, most importantly with Mary, but also with his friends. Mary has learned the signs and symptoms of hypoglycemia and knows what to do: usually it is an effective load of sugar, rarely a call to 911. This partnership extends to his friends or anyone who spends time with him. Fortunately, Rick has not hidden his diabetes from others as some patients do. If you spend time with Rick, you need to know he has diabetes and it is even prudent to have a basic understanding of hypoglycemia. I was reminded of this one evening when a small group of us were having dinner at Simon and Seafort's restaurant in Anchorage. After Rick had gone to the bathroom, an automatic timer went off in Mary's internal clock. "Tom, would you go and check on Rick, he has been gone too long." He was fine—most likely delayed on the way talking to a few of the many Alaskans who recognize him.

His positive, take-charge attitude has served him well in his public role and has been critical to the management of his diabetes. He understands his diabetes so well, he effectively manages his own treatment. He has discovered and describes well in this book his very earliest signs of low blood sugar, which many diabetics would miss. His very competent physician served as his coach early on, but now would best be described as a consultant. The results are impressive. After years of juvenile-onset, insulin-dependent diabetes, he has no complications. It has not prevented him from taking on any challenge whether it was in his public role, the variety of sports competitions he loves, or in other adventures and misadventures throughout his life.

Rick is a role model for diabetic patients, but also for those in public service. One will find his motivations are clear and altruistic. He has been driven by what he thinks will best improve the lives and well-being of those who have elected him to public office. His enthusiasm for life is infectious.

His positive attitude has carried him and others to achievements they never thought possible.

Who should read this book?

Definitely read this book if you have diabetes and want to achieve excellent control that allows you to live a fun-filled, challenging life. Rick gives you the recipe and tools for doing so.

Even if you do not have diabetes, you will have a basic understanding of a controllable disease that is reaching epidemic status secondary to obesity.

But these pages are for more than just diabetics. For Alaskans who lived through the '70s; '80s, and '90s it will bring back memories of the times we went through, the people with whom we were involved, and it gives us a peek behind the scenes at the "rest of the story."

For our children and grandchildren it is a primer on this dramatic time in the history of our young city and the experiences of their parents and grandparents.

Those outside Alaska will begin to understand the magic of Alaska, the can-do attitude of our citizens, our zest for life, our sense of adventure, and why we say to others, "It is North to the Future."

Thomas S Nighswander MD MPH

Professor of Family Medicine
Assistant Clinical Dean,
Alaska WWAMI Program
for the School of Medicine
University of Washington
Anchorage, Alaska

Acknowledgements

My profound thanks for the development of this book go to a number of people.

To my wife, Mary, who for 43 years has been at my side when I needed help. She's been supportive and concerned but never overly worried about my living with diabetes. She gave me good guidance in the organization and reorganization of this book and provided a clear sounding board for my ideas.

To our children, Nick, Rich, and Jen, who have given me joy, fulfillment, and the motivation to care for my health.

To my sisters, Rosanne Bader and Rochelle Breaux, and to my full extended family, including Rebecca Lindemann and Joe McKelheer, who have added so much to my life and to my motivation.

To my mom and dad who taught me, not with words, but by example.

To Asa Morton, my lifelong friend, whose first, long discussion with me about my diabetes got me started with the right attitude.

To Derek Gable, my lifelong friend and creative inspiration, for being a bountiful source of ideas for both the production and marketing of this book while always leaving me laughing at myself.

To Adele Morgan, a long-term Type 1 diabetic who continues to inspire Alaskans and Americans with her music and attitude toward diabetes and life.

To Susie Werner (now professor Susan Kieffer), who encouraged me through that first summer with diabetes, through written words, spoken words, and lots of hugs.

To Jeanne Bonar, my doctor for over 40 years, who guided and helped me throughout my journey with diabetes.

To my close friends, Dave Young, Rick Pollock, and Mike Johnson, who planted the seeds of this book by being so interested in what I had learned, and what I told them about foods.

To Rick Nerland, who read, reread, and corrected the chapters on Anchorage's Olympic bids to be sure I got them right.

To Fuller Cowell, Dr. Rob Benedetti, and Dr. John Mues, who all spent their time reading my manuscript long before it deserved even the briefest scrutiny.

To Flip Todd, who got me started on this long but fulfilling literary trail.

To Evan Swensen, my publishing consultant, who defined and clarified my path to a finished product.

To Marthy Johnson, who taught me how to bring life to my story.

And to all the thousands of volunteers and supporters who have so willingly embraced my projects and dreams for Alaska and helped give me the wonderful life that I've been blessed with.

Preface

This is the story of my life.
Not my whole life really, but my life with diabetes.

I was diagnosed with Type 1 diabetes in 1964 when I was 20 years old. I'm now approaching 70 and have lived with diabetes for nearly 50 years. Diabetes hasn't limited my activities, experiences, achievements, or happiness in any way and it doesn't have to limit yours, your children's or other loved ones'. It is, however, a thread that has run through my life every day and cannot be ignored.

Since I was first diagnosed more than 49 years ago, not a day has gone by when I haven't been aware of my diabetes—not every moment, of course, but frequently throughout every day. When I go to bed at night, when I wake up, when I eat, when I exercise, and when I'm starting an activity, I think about my blood sugar and I nearly always measure it at these times.

As a young man, I was especially sensitive to my diabetes when I was competing in football and basketball, when I was climbing mountains in Colorado for the Forest Service, and later working in the Alaska bush as a surveyor. As I've grown older, my sports have evolved to snow skiing, snowmobiling, waterskiing, wake-surfing, golf, tennis, and fishing, but each still requires me to be vigilant about my blood sugar levels.

Beyond sports there have been other times and events that required heightened vigilance, such as the moments prior to making each of the many hundreds of speeches I have given as chairman of Anchorage's—and later America's—Olympic Winter Games bids and as mayor of Anchorage, Alaska.

Someone just diagnosed with Type 1 or Type 2 diabetes may feel overwhelmed, but with a good attitude toward it, vigilance and testing will become part of your normal, accepted everyday life. Because of my open-to-learning approach to diabetes, I've learned firsthand which foods impact blood sugar and therefore insulin requirements the most. I've learned which foods contribute the most to weight gain and which foods don't. I haven't had to rely on others' opinions—some right and some wrong. I've learned by actual testing and graphing. I've learned the specific impact of different activities and the benefit of a simple, moderate exercise program. In other words, I've learned firsthand what it takes to live a healthy life.

Throughout my nearly 50 years as a diabetic, I can recall only one incident where I let my diabetes stop me from doing something I wanted to do. Four years ago, I backed out of an invitation from my friend, Steve Jones, to take a jet-skiing excursion through Prince William Sound, here in Alaska, in November. Some may graciously say that decision says more about my intelligence than it does about my fearfulness. In truth, I couldn't figure out how I could monitor my blood sugar levels through a dry suit while traveling at 30 miles per hour for hours at a time over 35-degree water in 20-degree air temperatures.

With the exception of that incident, I have kept the two promises I made to myself shortly after I was diagnosed with diabetes. The first was to never let diabetes keep me from doing anything I really wanted to do. The second promise was to *never complain about having diabetes*. Without exception, I have kept that second promise. This evolved into a positive attitude about having diabetes and a realization that it's not a burden. It's not a handicap. It's just my life. And so far it's been a long, healthy, productive, fun, and exciting life with diabetes.

Now I want to share my life experiences with you in the hope that it will help you understand your diabetes better and help you live healthier, better, and longer.

Prologue

I never expected to be here.

My wife, Mary, and I have lived in Anchorage for 41 years. Recently we built a second home on Finger Lake in the majestic Matanuska-Susitna Valley just 45 minutes north of Anchorage. Highlighting our view over the lake to the south is the landmark of the valley, the classically sharp and dominating Pioneer Peak. To the east is the glacier-packed Chugach Range, and to the west is the majestic Alaska Range with 20,320-foot Mount McKinley as its northern sentinel. To the north are the Talkeetna Mountains.

Our second summer in our lake home, Mary and I were hosting a family reunion for my side of our family—24 close relatives at our lake home and guesthouse for a week. More than anything else, it was the idea of family reunions that had motivated us to build our summer home here on Finger Lake. My sons, Nick and Rich, had helped me build a guesthouse on the property so everyone could be together for this and all the future reunions we dream of.

The summer patterns on Finger Lake are predictable. In tranquil morning hours, a half dozen or so small fishing boats dot the lake, fishing primarily for rainbow trout. On weekend afternoons the fishermen give way to water-skiers, wakeboarders and parents pulling their kids on brightly colored tubes that resemble floating armchairs. Beautiful summer evenings on the lake seem to last forever as Alaska's late-night twilight fades into the semi-darkness of midnight before light starts to reappear about 3 a.m.

It was a beautiful, sunny Alaska summer day in July, 2011, the first day of our reunion. In the early afternoon, Mary, my two sisters, Rosanne and Rochelle, and their husbands, Chuck Bader and Jay Breaux, and I sat on the deck reminiscing as we all watched our kids pulling our grandchildren on water skis and tubes. The shouts of the bigger children getting up on water skis for the first time and the squeals of the littler kids standing up on little water ski trainers offered happy interruptions of our conversation. It was such a joy watching our own children, now as young parents, encouraging and celebrating their children's achievements just as we had done with them thirty or more years before.

Earlier that morning Mary and I had taken our daughter, Jen, and her husband, Andy Scott, and their two little ones, Lily and Boden, our first grandchildren, out on our fishing boat. It's a simple, 8-by-16-foot pontoon boat with deck chairs and plenty of room to move around—a pleasant way to fish for the nice-size rainbow trout that populate our lake.

Lily was nearly five years old and Boden was coming up on three. We were all hoping they'd catch their first fish that morning. But I knew at their age if it didn't happen in the first five minutes they'd be ready to go home for Oreos and milk. I anchored at my favorite fishing hole. We

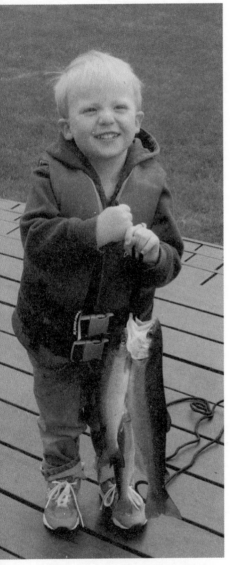

Boden struggles to hold up his first day's catch in Alaska. Caught with his Spiderman pole.

baited up Lily's Barbie fishing pole and Boden's Spiderman pole—and waited. I recollect it was only a few minutes but it seemed much longer when suddenly Boden's pole started jerking. A rainbow had grabbed his bait. We all started shouting and cheering. By our reaction, he knew it was something special. As we all cheered and encouraged him to reel it in, I glanced down at Lily, silently holding her immobile pole but barely holding back tears. I got down on one knee to console her and at that very moment her Barbie pole dived hard—another rainbow. Our grandkids both had their first fish on.

With all the cheering and yelling as both little kids worked at landing their fish, it was my turn to try to hold back tears. It was a precious moment—made much more precious because there had been a time in my life when I never expected to experience a moment like this. I never expected to live long enough to have grandkids. In fact, a few doctors had told me as much.

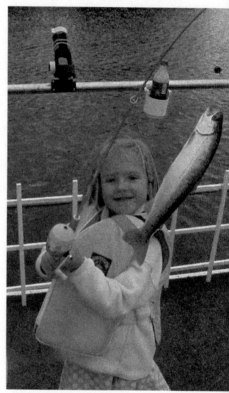

Lily proudly displays her first fish. Caught on her Barbie pole.

When I was diagnosed as a Type 1, insulin-dependent diabetic in 1964, the prognosis was pretty grim. Some basic forms of insulin were available, but no insulin pumps, no self-testing of blood sugar, and no real understanding of why diabetics frequently lost their limbs, lost their eyesight, experienced kidney failure, and died at a much earlier age than non-diabetics.

I remember one doctor telling me that by the time I was 40 years old, I could expect to have at least one of those major problems and maybe all four. I was 20 then and 40 seemed an eternity away. Forty was *old* to my way of thinking and so what if I had to walk with a cane or had kidney failure. I had a life to live—at least for 20 more years. Now here I am coming up hard on 70, enjoying grandkids, and still competing in sports—still snow-skiing, waterskiing, golfing, and learning new sports such as wakeboarding and wake-surfing.

In the summer of 2011, I was wakeboarding with two of my closest friends, Dave Young and Rick Pollock. Rick was driving my Mastercraft ski boat, which was bouncing through wakes caused by other boats, when the front of my wakeboard suddenly caught a wake and dove hard. I hit the water face and chest first with my feet solidly strapped into the bindings of the board. When I surfaced, I couldn't take a full breath. Each partial breath I sucked in felt like an arrow piercing my chest. Dave and Rick helped me back onto the boat and back to the dock.

Though every movement hurt, I had always told my boys to "shake it off and work through it" when they got hurt. So I did just that. But two days later the pain was so great that I decided to go to the emergency room at Providence Hospital in Anchorage. I walked in, told the receptionist what had happened, and filled out a simple admission form. She read the form and called back to an emergency room doctor while I waited at the counter. "Doctor, I've got a well-dressed, sixty-seven-year-old gentleman here who thinks he broke his ribs—wakeboarding." She paused for a moment, listening to his response, then said, "Yes, sixty-seven." "Yes, wake-boarding." Another pause. "His last name is Mystrom." Pause again. "Okay I'll ask him." She turned to me. "Are you related to the former mayor?" "Sort of," I replied. "I am the former mayor."

When I left the emergency room with the confirmation that I had at least one broken rib, the doctor smiled and said, "Don't take this wrong, Mr. Mayor, but you've made my day."

Two years prior to that incident I had taken a stress test at the suggestion of my doctor. My results equated to "an active 42-year-old"—about 23 years younger than my chronological age at the time. With all the grim predictions and lack of technology at the time of my original diagnosis, how did I get here? How was I able to live such an active, bold, productive, and fun life with diabetes? Why am I so healthy after nearly 50 years with diabetes? And why do I now believe I can live actively and well for many more years?

This is my story. I truly hope and believe it will help you or your loved ones live happier, healthier, and longer.

You can't always choose the road you will take in your life but you can choose whether you will walk on the shady side or the sunny side of that road.

—Anonymous

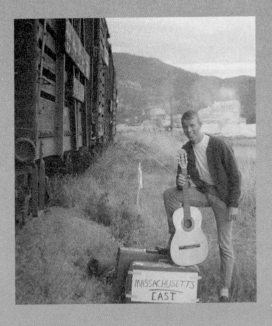

Hitchhiking and riding the rails on my way from California back to the University of Colorado in the summer of 1964. My traveling buddy, Doug Moore, was heading to Massachusetts.

Chapter 1

A Life-Changing Diagnosis

You've Got Diabetes

I'll never forget that day. It was a Friday afternoon in July 1964, a beautiful summer day in Boulder, Colorado. The morning was clear and sunny. I remember noticing that puffy, grayish cumulus clouds had rolled in by midafternoon. I was playing tennis with my girlfriend, Susie Werner, behind the Harvest Manor Apartments alongside Boulder Creek, just down the hill from the Colorado University campus. I think I was winning but likely just barely, knowing what a good athlete Susie was.

Life was good. I was a healthy, athletic 20-year-old with all the feelings of invulnerability that came with the confidence and testosterone that coursed through my body. Both Susie and I were attending summer school classes at CU. She was a recent summa cum laude graduate of Allegheny College in Pennsylvania and working on a PhD in astro-geophysics at CU, and I was an undergraduate trying to correct a few flaws in my modest academic transcript.

I was 6 feet 3 inches tall and weighed a lean 175 pounds, and I seemed to be always hungry and getting thinner. I didn't think any more of my continual hunger than I did of the fact that I went to the bathroom frequently. I think I just blamed that on Coors.

But that afternoon, my life changed forever. I had just had a physical exam and had some blood work done a few days before as required for my continuation in Air Force ROTC. The examining doctor, Richard Daarud, had been most complimentary about my physical condition. He was certain that the routine blood work would confirm his visual assessment that America would want me fighting on our side if that little conflict in Vietnam ever got bigger. He was wrong.

I was at the service line ready to serve to Susie when I looked up and saw my roommate, Rick Arkus, another fun-loving student of modest academic achievement, running across the lawn.

His face showed the thrill of someone who had a scoop, but realized that his excitement shouldn't overshadow the potential gravity of the message. His effort to meld those reactions failed miserably. The result was an inappropriate, excited laugh. "Dr. Daarud's office called and said you need to drop whatever you're doing and get in to see him now!" he said. "It can't wait. He'll stay at his office until you get there."

"I think something's wrong," he blurted, still trying to contain a smile that he knew didn't fit the occasion. "They wouldn't tell you to come in right away on a Friday afternoon unless something is wrong." In the back of my mind I knew Rick was right. In short order, I changed into long pants, hopped into my '55 Chevy, and arrived at the doctor's office.

"What do you know about diabetes mellitus—or sugar diabetes?" Dr. Daarud asked. "Not much," I said. "A kid in my high school, Terry Behn, had it. He couldn't eat sweets and he had to take shots every day." "Well," he said, "You've got diabetes."

It hit me hard. I didn't eat any more candy or drink more pop than a normal American kid. (I would later learn that eating candy or drinking pop has nothing to do with getting Type 1 diabetes). I was always lean. I played sports year-round. How could this be true? What did it mean? Were my sports days over? And, of course, the scary question—would I have to give myself shots every day?

He proceeded to tell me that he was certain I had diabetes since my blood sugar was over 400 milligrams per deciliter (mg/dl) and that normal was 75 to 105. Nothing else, he explained, would cause my blood sugar to be that high. He also told me he was almost certain it was Type 1 diabetes because of my age and my good physical condition, but he wanted to give me a glucose tolerance test on Monday to confirm his conclusion. In the meantime, his nurse would give me a substantial shot of insulin to tide me over and he wanted me to be sure to eat a big meal as soon as I left his office.

He explained that the shot of insulin would allow all that sugar (glucose) in my bloodstream to be absorbed into my cells to provide the energy they needed to function. Without any insulin the glucose would simply stay in my bloodstream and eventually exit in my urine. That meant no energy would get to my cells and the sugar (energy) would just be shed through my urine. The consequence of that was that my cells could get energy only from what little fat I had stored on my body.

This was my introduction to three of the early symptoms of diabetes: high blood sugar, frequent urination, and sugar in my urine. A fourth symptom is low energy and feeling tired. I never had that symptom, which in retrospect leads me to believe that the onset of my diabetes had been sudden and occurred not long before it was diagnosed.

Before the nurse came into the examination room to give me the shot, Dr. Daarud told me to go to Colorado University's Norlin Library over the weekend and look up everything I could about diabetes, then write down every question I could think of. On Monday, as I took the glucose tolerance test, he would answer all the questions I had written down. It turned out to be an excellent way to introduce me to diabetes.

After he left, the nurse came in to give me the first of some 8,000 shots that I would be giving myself over the next 16 years before I got my insulin pump. She went through the usual routine, rolling up my sleeve, putting alcohol on the target site, and sticking the needle in my arm. She started pushing the plunger but it wouldn't go. Evidently she had hit a bone or some tough ligament that blocked the needle. She put both thumbs on the plunger, one on top of the other, and pushed hard. The hypodermic needle separated from the cylinder and insulin exploded all over my shirt. I looked down and saw the needle still sticking my arm and the empty cylinder in her hand. She looked at me and said, "Sorry, it usually goes a little smoother than that." I told her I hoped so or I'd be spending a lot of time washing shirts. Her second attempt worked just fine and I left the doctor's office with a big shot of insulin in my system and a lot to think about.

I pulled up to my apartment but instead of going in I decided to take a walk along Boulder Creek and think about what was happening. I cried a little. I was worried but I don't recall being really afraid. I walked and struggled with the news for about an hour.

I was so wrapped up in trying to sort out my emotions that I had forgotten what Dr. Daarud had said about eating a big meal right away. The feeling was subtle at first, then more obvious. I felt a little weak, then slightly nervous. Then it dawned on me. I had a large dose of insulin going in and I was supposed to eat right away. I hadn't done that, so my blood sugar was dropping too low.

I ran across a field to a nearby restaurant, sat down at the counter and ordered a roast beef sandwich with mashed potatoes. Not the quickest-acting food to counteract a low blood sugar but I was smart enough, or lucky enough, to order a Coke instead of my usual milk. The Coke acted quickly enough to stop my falling blood sugar and keep me conscious until the rest of the food arrived.

Two things are memorable about that incident. First, I experienced my first low blood sugar, a feeling that I would have to be alert to every day for the rest of my life. Second, when I finished the meal, I actually felt satisfied. I didn't still feel hungry. Over the past weeks I'd felt hungry even after finishing a big meal.

Looking back I now realize what happened. The insulin the nurse had injected allowed my body to use the food I had just eaten. It allowed the glucose from the food going into my bloodstream to be absorbed by my cells instead of just collecting in my bloodstream and being eliminated in my urine. I felt stronger, more energetic, and for the first time in weeks I felt that my body had some fuel that would last me for at least a few hours.

Dr. Daarud had told me that the insulin his nurse would give me was fast acting and short-lived and would be in my system only three or four hours. And that I probably shouldn't eat too much the rest of the weekend because my body wouldn't be able to use food anyway.

The Start of a Positive Attitude toward Diabetes

That night instead of going to one of the many off-campus Friday-night parties in Boulder that were as spontaneous and prolific as summer dandelions, I decided to drive to Denver and hang out with my closest friend and confidant, Asa Morton.

Asa and I had roomed together our freshman year at CU and planned to room together again that coming fall. Asa was a chemistry student at CU; his dad, one of the most interesting people I've ever known, was a chemist. His mom, a lovely southern lady, had been a nurse in Tennessee before their family moved to Colorado. So Asa actually knew a bit about diabetes. More than I did, for sure, but that was easy since I knew practically nothing.

Asa had picked up from his dad the knack of being an interesting person to listen to, and from his mom the even more important characteristic of being interested in what the other person was saying. It made him a great conversationalist and friend: both interesting and interested.

We ended up that night at Davey's Diner in Lakewood, our favorite after-hours hangout. We had been talking about diabetes off and on all night and continued the discussion over our typical late-night meal of sausage and eggs for me and bacon and eggs for Asa. How two people could talk so much about something they knew so little about baffles me to this day, but we did. That night Asa said something that I'll never forget. It had a profound and positive impact on how I dealt with diabetes and as a result a huge, positive impact on my life in general.

I took a sip of the first cup of coffee I'd ever had without sugar. It was an almost pleasant surprise. "This isn't too bad."

Asa's reaction was quick and to the point. "That's exactly why you've got the right personality to deal with diabetes." "What are you talking about? What's the right personality to deal with diabetes?" "That's it, the coffee without sugar. You've already accepted it. That's what I'm talking about. You've got such a positive attitude about life, you're going to do fine with diabetes."

Nearly 50 years later as I reflect on that comment, I realize that more than anything else, more than eating right, exercising, being active, it's a positive attitude toward dealing with diabetes that stands alone as the single biggest contribution to my healthy, happy, productive life with diabetes.

A Promise Made

I spent quite a bit of time that weekend researching diabetes and talking to my family in California. My mom and dad were very concerned, sympathetic, and supportive and my two sisters, Rosanne and Rochelle, were very interested, supportive, and positive. I must have inherited the same positive-attitude gene both my sisters had or maybe just learned from their actions as we grew up together. My girlfriend, Susie, who was with me constantly that summer, was also very encouraging, caring, and thoughtful.

Asa's comment that I would do fine with diabetes stuck with me. That comment, combined with the support of my parents, my sisters, and Susie was critical in developing a positive attitude about diabetes. Shortly after that I made a promise to myself that I would never complain about having diabetes.

From that point on, I would look at diabetes not as a major problem but just as my life. I told myself that it was just like brushing my teeth in the morning. I would just wake up, give myself a shot, and forget about having diabetes. Well, it wasn't quite that simple. Once you brush your teeth, you can forget about it for a while, but once you give yourself a shot of insulin, you forget about it only at your peril.

I spent a lot of time thinking about my promise never to complain about having diabetes. As a young boy growing up, I hadn't been very good about keeping promises to myself or to God. My promises were often made when I'd say my prayers at night. Most often they involved pledges not to kill any more ants or spiders or shoot any more frogs if I would get an A on the homework paper I had rushed through or on a test I hadn't studied for.

I distinctly remember when I was 10 years old promising God that if I made the Little League all-star team I wouldn't draw airplanes during sermons ever again. I didn't think I'd have much of a chance to make it because 10-year-olds rarely did. The next morning I found out that I had made the all-star team. But I figured that decision must have been made before my prayer the night before so that promise probably didn't count.

But the promise never to complain about having diabetes I have kept without fail. To this day I believe it was the most important promise I have ever made with regard to my health. Over the years, many little problems such as tangles in my pump cords, forgetting my tester, or slightly underestimating or overestimating insulin needs all could have been sources of frustration. But somehow they never were. I attribute that to my promise never to complain.

That Monday I went back to Dr. Daarud's office to take a glucose tolerance test. It's really a simple test. I was given a large container of what tasted like a sweet, noncarbonated cola drink and told to drink about four ounces every 15 minutes. Also every 15 minutes a nurse took a blood sample and labeled it with the time taken. This process continued for three or four hours. The blood was sent to a laboratory to be tested for blood sugar (glucose) content and then graphed.

The pattern for a non-diabetic is a quick rise in blood sugar level and then an equally quick drop back to normal as soon as the insulin sent by the pancreas to the bloodstream begins working. The pattern for a diabetic starts with a quick rise but then continues up because the pancreas doesn't produce insulin that allows the sugar to be absorbed through the blood-vessel walls and into the cells for use by the body. The glucose just stays in the bloodstream. The blood sugar gets higher and higher. Some spills out in the urine but none is available for use by the body for energy, for storage, and for life itself.

As Dr. Daarud had promised, he came into the room where the test was being administered and began answering the three pages of questions I had written on a yellow tablet. It was a good learning exercise and a great start to understanding diabetes. Dr. Daarud made it very clear that with diabetes more than any other chronic disease, it was the patient who would control his or her own destiny and health. His philosophy was that a doctor could guide and advise me but it was up to me to make my own health.

Three days later results of the glucose tolerance test came back. It confirmed both what Dr. Daarud had concluded and what I had accepted. I had Type 1 diabetes.

*How full a life that I must
live, so much to learn,
so much to give.*

—Rick Mystrom (1964)

One of the many
motivational thoughts
I wrote to help me get
through the first few
months with diabetes.
Not much in the way
of poetic value but
the message has stuck
with me.

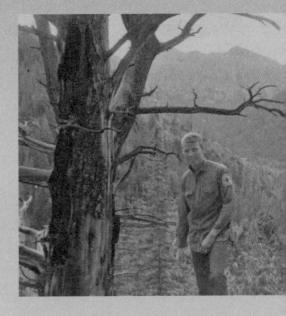

Climbing Mt. Elbert, Colorado's highest
mountain, with Asa, who took
the photo.

Photo courtesy of Asa Morton

Chapter 2

My Early Years with Diabetes

Managing Diabetes before Self-Testing

I began giving myself insulin shots soon after the results of the glucose tolerance test came back. Based on Dr. Daarud's recommendation I began giving myself a single shot of long-lasting (about 24–36 hours' duration) insulin called protamine zinc insulin (PZI). But without the ability to test my own blood sugar, I really had no idea how it was working and what my blood sugar levels were. What I did know was that after I began taking insulin, I felt better, I had more energy, and I began gaining weight. My weight went from a lean 175 pounds to a more muscular 190 pounds in a matter of three or four months because now my body could use the food I was eating. The insulin allowed the glucose in my bloodstream to be absorbed into my cells instead of just collecting in my blood and exiting in my urine.

During that first summer with diabetes I had some—but not a lot—of discussions with Susie about the predicted short life span I thought I was facing. I don't recall specifically telling myself I had to work harder and faster than my peers because my life would be shorter but I think the idea emerged in conversations once in a while. Looking back and trying to conjure up specifics of 50-year-old conversations is like trying to identify a bird by looking through binoculars backwards. You can tell it's a bird but the details have disappeared.

Fortunately, I saved a notebook of thoughts, verses, and poems I wrote to encourage and motivate myself that bring light to my hazy, uncertain recollection of my feelings of 50 years ago. One such thought appears as an epigraph at the start of this chapter. It tells me that I was focused on leading a full life. My inference from this distant retrospective is that working hard to compensate for an anticipated shorter life was a part of my thought process.

The notebook also contains some poems Susie wrote to me to encourage me to focus and persevere. The opening verse of one poem titled, "Find a Star, Young Man" appears as an epigraph at the start of chapter 11.

College and the Forest Service

Between the time I was diagnosed with diabetes in 1964 and the time I graduated from the University of Colorado in 1968, I continued an active lifestyle. I pitched for the best team in the city of Boulder's top fast-pitch softball league and played every year on competitive intramural football and basketball teams, winning a couple of all-school championships.

I was also mostly broke. My roommate and close friend, Art Horn, and I worked part-time washing dishes at a high-end steak house called the Red Lion. This wasn't as bad as it sounds since a lot of customers left large pieces of unfinished steak on their plates. Art and I tossed the bigger leftover pieces into a paper bag with the edges rolled down, which we kept about 12 feet away in a corner near the area where we stood clearing and washing plates. We competed with each other on a "shots-made percentage." When we missed, we threw the steak away. We weren't going to eat a piece of meat that had been on the floor. The occasional piece of unfinished rare steak was a real find since we could cook it again at home and it would still be only medium rare.

Art and I ate a lot of steak that year but that habit of eating "used steak" also succeeded in ending what seemed like a pretty promising evening with a couple of cute girls we invited over to our apartment for dinner. They allowed as how they knew we didn't have much money and that they were very appreciative that we had spent so much to treat them to a steak dinner.

In admirable candor but foolish naiveté, Art explained that we really hadn't paid for the steaks but we worked at the Red Lion and for dinner that night we had recooked the best pieces that the customers had graciously left on their plates. Needless to say, the girls didn't finish their food but the evening was finished in short order with no after-dinner enjoyment.

During my junior year at CU, I worked at IBM's new assembly plant in Boulder. I worked 20 hours a week from 5 to 9 p.m. Monday through Friday. At two dollars per hour, my gross was $40 per week and my net after taxes was $36.20. I didn't eat steak that year but I could at least buy hamburgers at McDonald's for 15 cents (17 cents for a cheeseburger) along with milk for 10 cents.

During my senior year, I'd show up periodically at the student employment office looking for part-time work. One day in late spring, I hit it big—$12 an hour—as a model for Gerry Backpacks. When they offered me the job, I had visions of climbing in the Colorado Rockies looking rough and rugged with one of their backpacks loaded with fake provisions. But that wasn't to be. They were looking for a model for their baby carriers. But for 12 bucks an hour, I would have carried the mom as well as the baby. Actually I did quite a bit of work for them, which carried me over until I started my summer job.

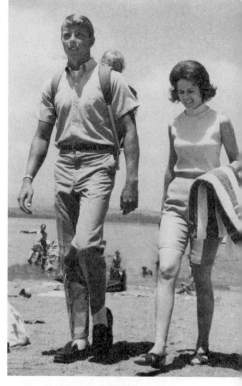

I thought I'd be modeling mountaineering backpacks. Instead I ended up modeling shopping-center baby packs. But at $12 an hour, I didn't complain.

Photo courtesy of Gerry Backpacks

My summer jobs were always enjoyable. One summer I was a lifeguard at the Harvest House Hotel pool in Boulder, where my job was to keep an eye on all the University of Texas coeds who traveled to Boulder every summer with their families to escape the Texas heat. I'm

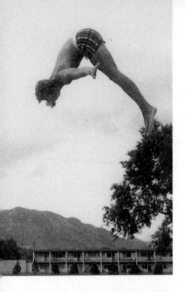

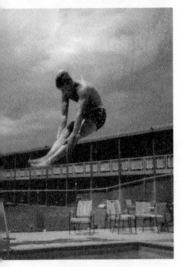

Practicing diving
on a break from my
lifeguarding duties.

proud to say that I took my job very seriously and not a single coed drowned during my watch, though a few tried convincingly to do so. I suspect they enjoyed the standard lifeguard cross-chest carry to the shallow end as much as I did.

Most summers during my college years I worked as a surveyor's assistant for the U.S. Forest Service in the mountains of Colorado and on the plains of Wyoming. Each June after finals, I'd load the trunk of my '55 Chevy with my summer necessities— Levis, T-shirts, flannel shirts, boots, and a couple boxes of books which, despite my self-promise to read them, I mostly just carried around in the trunk of my car.

The crews I was on did topographical survey-ing—defining the height and location of mountains for future topographical maps. It was a wonderful job that required the physical stamina to climb 12,000- and 13,000-foot peaks with packs filled with surveyor's instruments, as well as a 6-volt car battery to power them. When we got to the tops of the peaks, we needed a precise touch on the instruments and the mathematics background to use trigonometry to calculate the height and location of surrounding mountain peaks based on triangulation.

I worked most summers for a terrific person and good civil engineer by the name of Hank Masonier. He and his sweet wife, Eileen, kind of adopted me during those summers in the small Colorado towns. Hank taught me a little about surveying and a lot about life. I'm not so sure that I'm a better surveyor because of Hank but I know for sure that I'm a better person because of him. We were so wrapped up in philosophical, religious, and political discussions that I sometimes lost track of the tasks at hand. So if you ever find any mountains in Colorado that aren't where they're supposed to be, it's probably my fault.

As I reflect on those days in the mountains of Colorado and on the plains of Wyoming, I'm astounded that I did not carry some kind of sugar or candy in my pocket at all times. Now, I would never be out in the woods or the "bush" as we call it in Alaska, without my ever present small packets of Skittles. The Halloween-size packets of Skittles are the best and most convenient insurance against low blood sugar that I've found. They're loaded with sugar. They're fast to absorb and they're convenient to carry. The small packages are sufficient for all but the most extreme low blood sugars and I can always choose to carry two for additional insurance.

I never did have any severe low blood sugar reactions during my Forest Service days in Colorado or Wyoming. I'm sure that was because my blood sugar in those days was probably pretty consistently high. Because of the absence of low blood sugar reactions, I put myself in some pretty dangerous situations—hours away from any help and often near or at the top of mountain peaks.

Trapped on Rattlesnake Ridge

I survived my summers in the mountains and plains without anything worse than spending one night lost in the San Juan Mountains, north of Del Norte, Colorado and another night perched in the dark for eight hours on a flat-topped, kitchen-table-sized, four-foot-high rock on a hundred-yard-long outcropping known as Rattlesnake Ridge in eastern Wyoming.

That afternoon, with no rattlesnakes in sight, I had built a 12-foot-high signal made out of 12-foot-long 2-by-2s, and red and white flagging. I centered the signal at the top of the ridge so the engineers, who were 10 to 15 miles away, could shoot it with a sophisticated transit the next day to determine the ridgetop's exact location and altitude. But by trying to get it finished before sundown, I waited too long and got myself in trouble.

It was getting darker and cooler. That wasn't a problem I thought. I'd finish up and could still find my Jeep in the dark. I had to get the signal up. I was so wrapped up in finishing before the dusk turned to dark that at first I didn't notice that rattlesnakes had started emerging from their shaded cover. They weren't yet close to me so I kept working. But it subtly and seemingly quickly happened. The next time I looked up, snakes were all around me. Moments later, in the gathering darkness I could barely see them. I had a semiautomatic, 22-caliber Winchester but no flashlight. I thought if I shot a few in the remaining dusk maybe the rest would panic and disappear. I shot three of them but found out that rattlesnakes don't panic. They just get agitated. Within the minutes it took me to gather my tools and think about getting out of there, I couldn't see them at all.

Could I walk through that minefield of rattlesnakes in the dark to my Jeep about 3 miles away or should I climb up on the small, flat-topped rock and hunker down for the night? If I stepped on just one snake it would cause all of them to respond with aggression. I chose hunkering down.

For a while, I tried sitting cross-legged on the rock but thought I could easily fall off if I fell asleep. I didn't have a belt so I couldn't attach myself to the signal I'd built. I tried lots of positions—none very good. I finally leaned against the signal post and pulled my legs up to my chest. That was okay for a while. As I sat there, I listened to the quiet, scary sound of hundreds of snakes slithering around me. This was no time to have a low blood sugar reaction.

It was a long, cold night. Though the temperature probably didn't get much below 55 degrees Fahrenheit, my body temperature seemed to drop gradually over the hours. Fortunately I had a light jacket just in case any sudden summer rain and wind came up but it was very difficult to keep warm just sitting on a rock for what was to be about eight hours. At first I stood up and moved my legs up and down but quit that when it got completely dark. I kept visualizing falling of the rock and dancing around in the dark on the heads and bodies of surprised, angry rattlers. The top of the rock was big enough that I could curl up into a ball and try to sleep. Minutes crawled by as I tried in vain to read my watch.

When the sky in the east began to lighten with the impending sunrise, I could see what I had been hearing for about nine hours: more than a hundred rattlers within sight and still milling around in the cool of the summer morning. For about two hours I tried different methods of counting them so I could relay the story with some degree of accuracy to the rest of the crew, who by that time had come out looking for me. My attempt at counting gave me something to do and helped the last couple of hours pass faster.

By about 10 a.m. the snakes began moving westward toward the shady side of the ridge and protection from the coming heat of the eastern sun. Within about 10 minutes the eastern slope of the ridge was clear of any visible snakes. I got down from my perch and walked unimpeded to my Jeep. By the time I got to my vehicle, other crew members had found it and were preparing to head out on a now unnecessary search for me.

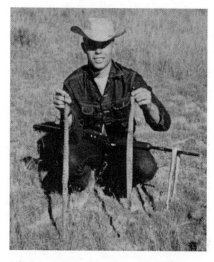

After a night on Rattlesnake Ridge, my boss's only comment to me was, "We've got work to do. Let's get going."

The Poster That Changed My Life

One typically warm and sunny summer morning back in Boulder, Colorado, I was scheduled to meet my girlfriend, Marcy Tonish, in front of the Norlin Library on campus. I waited a few minutes for her but knowing she was in a class with a professor who was often indifferent to the class-ending buzzer, I decided to head toward her classroom. When I got there the class

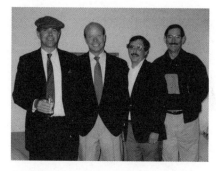

My four closest friends from college at a reunion forty years later. *Left to right:* Art Horn, me, Steve Kinney, and Asa Morton.

was still in session so I hung around outside for a few minutes. It was there that I saw a poster on the wall that said "Surveyors Wanted. Alaska."

Since I had no idea what I was going to do with a degree in political science, I applied for the job and got it. I graduated in June and soon after headed for Alaska. I often wonder what my life would have been like if that professor hadn't let his class out late. That little serendipitous event led to a wonderful life for me and I hope a better life for many Alaskans.

"You've got a full and exciting life ahead of you, Rick. Go live it."

—Dr. Richard Daarud (1968)

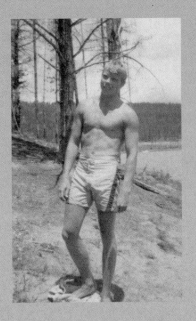

Within months after I started taking insulin, I gained about 15 good, solid pounds. My body was now able to use the food I ate.

Photo courtesy of Sally Baker

Chapter 3

A Summer in Alaska

Graduation Night

The last day of my classes at the University of Colorado was June 5, 1968—
an unforgettable day but not for the usual reasons. My graduation party at
the apartment I shared with my close friend Art Horn started early and
continued late. It was about 2 a.m. when I saw a couple of guys carrying
our old black and white TV from our run-down apartment. I yelled above
the blasting Beatles hit, "Yellow Submarine," "Hey, where are you guys
going with that?" I started to walk toward them. One of them yelled back,
"Bobby Kennedy's been shot." Others heard him. Within seconds someone
reached the volume control of the music and cut it. The partygoers started
streaming out to other apartments or to their cars.

The party was instantly transformed from loud, celebratory chaos to
quiet disbelief and sad, sober questions. Was he still alive? Who shot him?
Why? We learned he was shot at the Ambassador Hotel in LA shortly
after he had won California's Democratic primary for president of the
United States. Our neighbors, who were taking the TV down to their
apartment away from the noise so they could find out what was happening, brought it back to our now quiet apartment, so we could watch the
coverage there.

I remember my roommate, Art Horn, Asa Morton, and I slouching on our old, beat-up, faded tan sofa, sharing in stunned disbelief the fact that from the time we had graduated from high school to our college graduation night, President John F. Kennedy, Martin Luther King, and now Robert Kennedy had all been shot and killed.

Art and I had been together in a Jeep on the plains of eastern Wyoming when we heard that President Kennedy had been shot. We had listened incredulously to our two-way radio. Not too many moments later, we heard these unforgettable words, "The president is dead."

We stopped what we were doing and headed for the nearest town, Lusk, Wyoming to see if we could get any more news. The first building we saw as we drove into that silent little town was an automotive repair garage. Through the open garage door we saw three men gathered in front of a small black and white TV. They were hard-working, strong-looking men. They wore dirty coveralls and had greasy, dirty hands from their work—the kind of grease and dirt that will never go completely away. We pulled up to the garage in our government Jeep and walked in. They didn't even turn around until we got very close to them. When the guy closest to us finally turned around, he had little rivulets of tears trickling down both cheeks. We didn't say a word. Neither did they. We just stood silent and watched.

Just two months before Bobby Kennedy's assassination, Asa and I and three other friends—Doug Jackson, Jim Laurie, and his girlfriend, Judy— had been on our way back to Boulder from a spring-break road trip to Las Vegas when we heard that Martin Luther King Jr. had been shot and killed. The startling sadness of that event was softened by five friends being together in a car. We talked about what Dr. King had done for America. We talked about his great, compelling speeches. But mostly we talked about what was happening to America.

Now, Asa, Art, and I were together again during the third assassination of an American leader in less than five years. These events marked the 1960s as the most tumultuous American decade in the 20th century. Those sudden and unexpected tragedies were defining times in the lives of most Americans who will never forget where they were or who they were with at those indelible moments.

I didn't know it then, but those series of events would change my life dramatically and lead me into politics.

A Summer in Alaska

Before I left Boulder, I met one last time with Dr. Daarud. At that appointment, he commented on how healthy I looked since I had started taking insulin. His exact words were, "You're certainly developing a powerful-looking physique, Richard." He favored calling me Richard since that was also his name and he commented that he had grown to think of me a little like a son as well as a patient. We talked about my going to Alaska and working in the bush (Alaskan term for the backcountry). He gave me the assurance that having diabetes should in no way stop me from doing that. I remember him saying, "Rick, you've got a full and exciting life ahead of you. Go live it." At that point, with my limited understanding of diabetes, had he discouraged me from going, I probably would not have taken the job and never ended up living in Alaska.

One week later I was on my way to Juneau, Alaska to begin a job with the Bureau of Public Roads as a summer employee doing preliminary surveying for roads to be built. In reality, preliminary surveying means you're the first ones through a backwoods area that may someday be a roadbed. It's really more cutting brush and trees and creating sight lines than it is surveying. It was every bit as physically demanding but not nearly as complex or mentally challenging as the topographic and cadastral surveying I had done in Colorado and Wyoming.

The day after I arrived in Juneau and checked in with the Bureau of Public Roads office, I was sent down to Ketchikan for a month to help a crew down there. Ketchikan is the southernmost town in Alaska and its geography can best be described as a northern rainforest. Its industry then was fishing and logging. Deer Mountain backdrops the town and the residents refer to it as the world's largest weather vane: if you can't see the mountain, it's raining. If you can see the mountain, it's about to rain.

The town is on Revillagigedo Island and our job was to identify and cut sight lines for a road from Ward Cove to the George Inlet on the other side of the island from Ketchikan. On the flight to Ketchikan, I met a sweet, pretty Alaska Airlines stewardess, Kathy Jeleski. I was already beginning to appreciate Alaska's beauty.

My First Severe Low Blood Sugar Reaction

Since the work in Ketchikan involved a 4- or 5-mile walk-in every day, often using machetes to cut devil's club and other noxious brush as well as using chain saws to cut trees for sight lines, I decided that I didn't want to use a long-lasting insulin that would be continuously putting insulin into my bloodstream. I figured, correctly as it turned out, that it would be safer to give myself two shots of quick-acting, regular insulin each day; one in the morning before breakfast and one in the evening before dinner.

My logic was that if I ate a sufficiently big breakfast, it would cover the insulin going into my system for the next few hours; by midday, there wouldn't be any insulin going in so the danger of a low blood sugar episode out in the woods would be minimal. My system worked. I had only one "severe" low blood sugar episode during my time working out of Ketchikan.

That incident happened on a Monday after I had taken a shot of long-lasting protamine zinc insulin late Sunday morning the day before. Since I had Sundays off and was always in town, I didn't worry about having long-lasting insulin going into my system. But what I didn't realize then was that the long-lasting insulin I had taken on Sunday would continue into my body for 36 hours. It was still going in on Monday and would combine with my usual morning shot of quick-acting insulin. Together the two shots were too much when combined with all the glucose I was burning fighting my way through the brush.

By midmorning I was starting to get weak and a little disoriented. I knew what was happening and told my partner and buddy, Ricardo Roybal from New Mexico, that I needed to stop and eat the sandwich I had made for lunch. My sandwich didn't feel like it was sufficient to bring my blood sugar up so he gave me his sandwich too. Together they brought my blood sugar up and I was starting to feel better but foolishly I decided to continue working without any food or drinks in my pack or my pockets.

After another couple of hours of fighting through the underbrush, I began once again to feel the unmistakable signs of low blood sugar. We were 5 or 6 miles from our Jeep, which was parked at the end of the road about 15 miles out of town. I told Ricardo that we had to head back right away. I knew this was serious. I'd never been in this situation—low blood sugar and dropping and nothing to stop it with. I didn't really know what would happen if it got too low. About halfway back to the Jeep, I got too weak and confused to go on. I sat down. Ricardo sat down next to me. I started telling him what I had read about insulin shock and how I thought his best choice was to stay with me. If I lost consciousness and began to convulse, which is common with insulin shock, I had read that my body would start producing adrenaline which would trigger the release of glycogen from my liver. That would raise my blood sugar. I thought I would regain consciousness within an hour or so. Then we could continue out to the Jeep. At that time I had not yet experienced severe or extreme hypoglycemia so I was relying only on what I had read.

But as we sat talking, we both looked up at about the same time. From that low vantage point we saw the underside of the bushes on the uphill side of the trail loaded with salmonberries (a yellowish, raspberry-like berry). They weren't very ripe but there were a lot of them and they were my only hope to avoid a seizure and unconsciousness.

Ricardo started picking the berries furiously and brought me a handful within about 30 seconds. While I consumed those as quickly as I could, he brought me more. Because they weren't fully ripe, they didn't taste sweet and I had some doubts about whether I was getting any sugar from them. But after consuming about four or five handfuls within about five minutes, I could feel they were working and about 15 minutes later I felt strong enough to continue walking out.

I knew I wasn't out of danger yet because I didn't know how much residual insulin was still going in and we were a few miles from the Jeep. As we negotiated the final miles along the narrow trail through the brush, I didn't feel really strong but I was oriented and thinking clearly so I knew, although my blood sugar was still low, it wasn't dangerously low.

When we got to the Jeep, I told Ricardo, "Step on it. I need to get someplace to get a candy bar or Coke fast." Well, that was all the encouragement he needed. He pushed that Jeep hard along the narrow, winding dirt road. Dust billowed from the back tires sliding loose on nearly every turn.

We got to a small store in about 20 minutes and Ricardo ran in. He came out seconds later with a Coke and a candy bar. Within minutes after I drank the Coke, my blood sugar started coming up and I felt stronger and more coherent. I also ate the candy bar, which was probably overkill.

Categorizing the Seriousness of Low Blood Sugar Episodes

In *The Johns Hopkins Guide to Diabetes*, Saudek, Rubin, and Shump (1997)[1] clearly describe the degrees of hypoglycemia (low blood sugar), and divide them into three stages:

> *Mild Hypoglycemia.* When you are mildly hypoglycemic, the symptoms are mainly physical: sweating, trembling, and so on. You can recognize them. You may notice that you aren't thinking as clearly as you usually do or that you aren't behaving quite normally, though others might not notice these subtle changes.

> Even mild hypoglycemia can be distressing, but most people don't find these episodes terribly upsetting.

> *Moderate Hypoglycemia.* When you are moderately hypoglycemic, you may become confused or act inappropriately, but you can still treat the low blood sugar yourself.

> *Severe Hypoglycemia.* When you are severely hypoglycemic, you are no longer able to self-treat. You are too confused to know what's going on. You may even fall into a coma or suffer a seizure.

---

[1] Saudek, C. D.; Rubin, R. R.; & Shump, C. S. (1997). *The Johns Hopkins Guide to Diabetes for Today and Tomorrow.* Baltimore: The Johns Hopkins University Press, page 68.

For the purposes of this book, I split up *severe hypoglycemia*. I continue to use that term to describe being unable to put your thoughts together to self-treat and needing someone else to help to get some form of sugar into your system. But I remove reference to a seizure or coma from that category and add a fourth category: *Extreme hypoglycemia.*

> *Extreme Hypoglycemia.* When you are extremely hypoglycemic you may suffer a seizure or a coma and require professional emergency help (paramedics or fire department) and/or transportation to an emergency facility.

I'll use these terms throughout this book to describe the stages of hypoglycemia (low blood sugar). Additional factors must also be considered. For example, "moderate hypoglycemia" with insulin and no food going into your system can become "severe hypoglycemia" very quickly. But "moderate hypoglycemia" with food going into your system faster than insulin is going in is not a problem. It's also important to note that throughout this book I'll use the terms *hypoglycemic* reaction and *low blood sugar reaction* interchangeably.

You can live an active and fulfilling life with diabetes just as I have. I had to learn from experience to avoid the dangers of extreme low blood sugar reactions. You can learn how to avoid them from this book and from my companion book, *The New Diabetic Lifestyle*. By applying what you learn in these two books you will be able to minimize or completely avoid these uncomfortable and sometimes dangerous reactions.

A Guide to Blood Sugar Levels and Reactions

Over the years I've learned that having a blood sugar level below the point where you are able to remain conscious is an emotionally draining and dangerous experience. If you can catch your declining blood sugar in time and bring it back up, it's like nothing happened. You feel normal within minutes. Between normal and extremely low is a continuum of blood sugar levels and impacts on your body and brain. Based on my 50 years of experience, I compiled the following guide to help insulin-dependent diabetics and their loved ones understand and cope with low blood sugars.

Symptoms of Low Blood Sugar by the Numbers

In the United States, blood sugar is measured by the term *mg/dl*, milligrams of glucose per deciliter of blood. So when you measure your blood sugar using any one of the scores of testers available, the number on your device is telling you the milligrams of glucose per deciliter of your blood at that moment.

Below are the low blood sugar symptoms that I've experienced at different levels over the past 30 years of self-testing. As you read these levels you will notice some overlap. For example 70mg/dl could fit in either the first or the second category. This overlap is simply because these numbers are not intended to imply a specificity that cannot be felt. In other words, nobody can feel the difference between 70mg/dl and 71mg/dl. These numbers are intended to be a general guide and may differ slightly between individuals.

105 mg/dl down to 70 mg/dl — These are ideal levels. Everything feels fine. I can think clearly. My coordination is good. I sleep well. I can hit a golf ball straight, though normal blood sugar doesn't guarantee that I always will.

70 down to 60 — I can begin to feel these lows. I notice weakness if I'm doing anything strenuous like climbing hills or stairs, lifting, shoveling snow, playing tennis or similar activities. If I'm not doing anything strenuous, I may not feel anything abnormal.

60 down to 55 — These are the levels where I will feel weak even if I'm totally sedentary: reading, talking, watching TV and so forth. I feel less energetic and—as my kids would attest—a little irritable. These levels are not in themselves dangerous but the important issue is how fast your blood sugar is going down. If you don't have much insulin "on board"— in other words, going into your body—these levels are not emergencies, but if you do have insulin on board and no food going in, quick action is required.

55 down to 50 — At these levels I have difficulty completing complex thoughts. I'll get partway through explaining a thought and be unable to finish it. At that point I'll often stop and tell whoever I'm conversing with that my blood sugar is low and I need something with sugar—soft drink, candy, apple juice, or orange juice. At these levels I'm still thinking clearly enough to handle it myself.

The other symptom at these levels is a significant loss of motor skills. This is most obvious for me in the sport of golf. Other sports that require hand-eye coordination but not such detailed precision don't typically alert me to a low blood sugar problem as quickly as golf does.

I can recall times on the driving range when I was hitting the ball just fine—then out of nowhere I'd start mis-hitting balls—five, six, seven in a row—before it occurred to me to measure my blood sugar. I'd measure and usually find my blood sugar was in the 50–55 range.

When I'm playing golf, low blood sugars in this range manifest themselves in three or four terrible mis-hits in a row on the course. Now, I'm perfectly capable of two or three bad shots on a hole even if my blood sugar is normal so that's not always a reliable indicator. My regular golfing buddies, Dave Young, Rick Pollock, and Mike Johnson claim that they'll let me go with my blood sugar low for a couple of holes until I register a few double bogeys and they've made up some strokes on me.

50 down to 45 — At these levels of low blood sugar, I can't read a magazine, newspaper, or a book. The pages appear to have bright spots all over them that mask many of the words. I also begin to see bright flashes around the room. I quickly recognize the problem as well as the solution. I know I have to get something into my body as quickly as I can to raise my blood sugar. I can still figure out what I have to do and do it. I can solve things myself as long as Coke, juice, chocolate, or Skittles are handy.

It's also important to note that doing something very intense or competitive may mask symptoms at these or even lower levels. Waterskiing is a good example. When waterskiing I'm often focused, intense, and in very cold water. All those factors contribute to a fast drop in blood sugar levels. A number of times while waterskiing, I've gotten down to 50mg/dl without feeling it. Waterskiing in cold water in early spring in Arkansas once triggered an extreme low blood sugar that resulted in unconsciousness and an ambulance trip to a hospital emergency room.

45 down to 40 — At these blood sugar levels it's very difficult for me to help myself. I know something is wrong but I can't always figure out what's happening. My decision making is impaired. This is an urgent problem. Even when I figure out that I need something from the refrigerator, a number of times I've gone into the kitchen, opened the door and stood there in front of the open door just staring in and not knowing what to do or even why I'm looking into an open refrigerator.

At such times it's essential to call out to someone for help. For me it's usually my wife, Mary, who will quickly mix chocolate syrup with Coke and hand it to me. By that time I'm usually sitting on the floor or on a step with my head in my hands. The chocolate in the Coke makes the Coke flatter and easier to drink quickly. And quick is essential. At that point I don't worry about putting too much sugar in my body because the consequences of my blood sugar continuing down are so much more serious than the consequences of my blood sugar going up too much for a short period of time.

The confusion that results from this level and below is the very reason that it is so important that family and friends know what to do and how to help. They need to ask, "Are you okay?" "Do you need some sugar, a soft drink, or a candy bar?" Most of the time you'll have solved this problem before it gets to this stage. You will have felt your sugar getting lower and eaten or drunk something to raise your blood sugar, but if you haven't caught it in time, you need to count on your family or friends.

Even in a public place you need to ask someone for help before you get so confused you can't ask. I recall one time while I was mayor, I was driving in to City Hall and realized my blood sugar level was dangerously low and I needed something quickly. The City Market near downtown was on my route just a few blocks ahead. When I reached it I turned a hard left, parked my car, and walked quickly into the market. By that time, though, I was beyond the point of being able to find any soft drinks or help myself in any way. I stood near the entrance holding on to the edge of a display rack. The next person to walk in was a lady who stopped, put her hand on my arm and said "Are you okay?" "No," I said. "I need some sugar quick." She grabbed a Pepsi off a shelf about 10 steps away, opened it and had it in my hand in no time. Within two minutes or so my blood sugar had gone up enough for me to realize the crisis had passed. I thanked her but never got her name. So whoever you are, thank you again for realizing I needed help and helping.

A second episode requiring me to ask for help publicly happened at the Ryder Cup Golf Match at the Medinah Golf Club near Chicago in September 2012. I had traveled from Alaska to Chicago with 13 Alaskan friends to see the matches featuring the best American golfers vs. the best European golfers and to play some golf ourselves.

During the first day of the three-day contest, I had been watching the matches with three of my friends—Eldon Mulder, James Armstrong, and Craig Tillery. We had been moving around the course and watching the contest from various locations. By the end of the day we had been walking and standing for about 10 hours. That in itself is not a big deal, but the significance is that continual movement such as that for so many hours burns a lot of calories and brings down blood sugar much faster and more consistently than a normal day's activity for me. For lunch I'd eaten only a hot dog with half the bun—my typical habit when I eat hot dogs or hamburgers—and had only a bottle of water to drink. That wasn't much in the way of calories or blood sugar support for the amount of activity that day.

About 4 p.m. I could feel my blood sugar getting low but that wasn't a problem. I had a regular-size packet of M&Ms in my pocket along with my omnipresent Halloween-size packet of Skittles. I ate the full packet of M&Ms and felt confident that would bring my blood sugar up sufficiently until we stopped for dinner on the way back to the house we were renting.

As that day's matches ended at about 6 p.m., we began making our way with thousands of other spectators toward the buses which would take us to the Arlington racetrack, where all the cars were parked. Just as we exited the golf course, my blood sugar felt low again. I shouted to my friends to wait because I was going to test my blood sugar. It was 45 mg/dl and likely going down since I was continuously burning calories and using the glucose in my blood. But I still had my small packet of Skittles. I popped those in my mouth in hopes it would stop the drop in blood sugar as it almost always did. This time, however, it wasn't enough. The glucose I was burning overrode the input of sugar from the Skittles and by the time I got on the bus, my blood sugar was 40.

I knew my blood sugar was still going down because of the continuation effect of exercise. Blood sugar will typically continue down for up to a half hour after exercise or activity is complete. Eldon, who was sitting next to me on the bus, thoughtfully asked for a quick primer on what to do if I lost consciousness. I told him to just try to keep me from hurting myself if I had a seizure and have someone call 911. Then I stood up in the darkened bus and announced that I had diabetes and needed something sweet right away. A man a few seats in front of me had a half full bottle of Sprite, someone else passed me some Lifesavers, and a woman's voice behind me asked if pretzels would help. "They will," I said.

I drank the remaining Sprite, ate the Lifesavers and had some of the pretzels. Within minutes my blood sugar was up and everything was back to normal. It can be tough to do but sometimes you need to ask for help publicly. Do it without hesitation. People will help.

40 down to 30 — These levels are serious—and urgent. If you have insulin going in, you may be a minute or two from seizure and unconsciousness. You don't have time to measure your blood sugar. You just have to know the symptoms: confusion, brightness to the point you can't see well, inability to recognize your surroundings. At these levels I can't find the refrigerator; I can't find a door to get out of or into my house, I can't find a soft drink or candy in a grocery store, and I was once unable to find the door of a convenience store even as I stood in front of it.

You must understand the urgency at this blood sugar level. Don't wait. Act immediately. Call to anyone nearby to help you. Although I haven't had any extreme low blood sugars requiring medical help in the past 20 years, I have had a couple of close calls with my blood sugar below 40.

One early summer morning at our lake house, I woke up realizing my blood sugar was dangerously low. Based on the symptoms it was probably below 40. I walked out to the living room and shouted for Mary. But she was outside watering her flowers. It's a common early-morning enjoyment of hers and somehow I remembered that, but I couldn't find the door to get out to where I knew she was. This is a house that has seven doors leading outside and I couldn't find one. My brain was starved for glucose and was shorting out.

Everything was bright and confusing. I couldn't find the refrigerator. I stumbled across the door leading out to the garage and saw an unopened twelve-pack of Cokes in a cardboard container. I tried to figure out how to open the box along the perforated lines but couldn't. A Coke was exactly what I needed but I couldn't think clearly enough to just rip open the box. I put it down.

I wandered back into the living room and yelled again for Mary. No answer. I stumbled into our bathroom—nothing there. Then I weaved into our bedroom, where I had started four or five minutes before. There on my nightstand was a Coke and some chocolate syrup I always keep there. I sat on my bed weak and confused and alternated sips of Coke with the chocolate.

In a matter of minutes my blood sugar started to come back up. Within three or four minutes my blood sugar was high enough for me to walk into the living room, out the 12-foot-high doors that lead outside to the flowers on the south patio and tell Mary what had happened. Walking out the door to get help sounds simple but it's not. Not when your blood sugar is so low your brain can't function. You can look right at a door and still not see it.

If you catch the low blood sugar in time, as I did in this instance, you'll feel absolutely normal in a matter of minutes with no repercussions. If you don't catch it in time, you're in for a seizure, unconsciousness, and an ambulance ride to the hospital. That's no fun and is emotionally draining—not to mention the possibility of injury caused by falling (usually face first) during a seizure.

Below 30 — Only once have I been below 30 and still been conscious. That was about 20 years ago when I recall registering a 27 on my glucose meter. Hopefully you (or your diabetic child or loved one) will never get that low or lower but if you do, it's important to know what to expect.

If you, as an insulin-dependent diabetic, have your blood sugar drop into the 30s and have insulin on board but no food going in, your blood sugar is likely going to continue down until it gets into the 20s. At that level you will have a seizure and lose consciousness. From that point on you will be aware of nothing. No pain. No time awareness. No dreams. No memory—nothing. It's much like being under anesthesia, without medical supervision and with a seizure thrown in.

My experience with emergency medical technicians is that they are well trained in dealing with extreme low blood sugar situations. According to my wife, the first thing they'll do is test my blood sugar. They then put in an IV (intravenous drip) of what's colloquially called DW50. That's 50 percent dextrose and 50 percent water. That begins the process of bringing my blood sugar up.

Usually I don't begin to gain any awareness until I'm in the emergency room at a hospital. However, twice in longer ambulance rides I became semiconscious in the ambulance. In the emergency room I gradually become aware of people around me talking about me. Almost always the very first thing I remember is a doctor or a nurse saying, "He's starting to come around." My blood sugar starts approaching normal levels and things start to clear up very quickly for me. Within about 15 minutes I start having conversations with the doctor or nurse and within half an hour I'm ready to leave.

Twice I recall being injured in an extreme low blood sugar episode. Once I fell face first on the tile floor of a McDonald's restaurant and ended up with a black eye and a bruised nose. A second time my convulsions were so extreme that I herniated a disc in my back, which required an operation—successful, I'm pleased to report. That operation was in 1991 and I haven't had a back problem since.

Two years ago Mary and I took our preschool grandchildren, Lily and Boden, to Disneyland. Lily fell and scraped her knee so Mary took her to the little medical facility just off Main Street in the park while I stayed with Boden. While Lily was getting her scrape cleaned and bandaged, Mary asked the nurse what was the most common problem they dealt with. Without hesitation the nurse said, "Low blood sugar"—another illustration of the blood-sugar-lowering impact that continual walking will have.

What If No Emergency Help Is Available

Periodically someone will ask me what happens if no medical help or other help is available. If you're on your own and unconscious, then what happens? I've had only one experience with that situation. My eight-year-old son, Richard, and I were at the Golden Horn Lodge, a fishing lodge in western Alaska, run by my friends, Bud and Holly Hobson. I had invited Doug Dicken, a friend and board member of my company to join us.

After our first day of fishing and a nice dinner, Rich and I headed up to our room for the night. I must have given myself too much insulin because sometime during that night my blood sugar went below the level that would allow me to remain conscious. I woke up about 5 a.m. on the floor with sore muscles, bruised elbows, and a knot on my head. I had experienced an extreme low blood sugar episode during the night and come back to consciousness without outside help.

The convulsion, as explained to me later, triggered the release of adrenaline which in turn released glycogen from my liver and brought my blood sugar back up. So even if you're out in the woods, the backcountry, or alone anywhere and you have a convulsion and lose consciousness, you will likely recover naturally. The danger, of course, is injury to yourself and/or exposure to the elements.

Extreme low blood sugar episodes are not to be taken lightly. They're emotionally difficult. They can be dangerous. And they scare the heck out of family members. So my advice to you is this: "Don't let it happen to you." It took me nearly 30 years to figure out the keys to avoidance. You'll learn how to avoid them in this book and in my companion book, *The New Diabetic Lifestyle*.

"Spectator Fans Three and Homers"

Shortly after my low blood sugar episode with Ricardo in the woods outside Ketchikan I had one of my most unique sports experiences ever. One Sunday while Ricardo and I were in our hotel room, I heard on the radio that a good fast-pitch softball team in Ketchikan was playing a team from the USS *Tortuga*, a navy ship docked for a few days at the harbor. Having been a fast-pitch pitcher during my college years in Boulder and later in Southern California, I was always interested in seeing how pitchers in other states performed. My reputation had been lots of speed and not so much control. In fact more than once I threw a riser over the catcher, the ump, and almost over the backstop. My curve escaped so frequently that the on-deck batter was often as worried about getting hit as the batter was. But when I found my groove I could be unhittable.

I decided to walk up to the game to check out the quality of the pitchers. It was a warm, sunny day in Ketchikan so I put on my usual "hanging-out clothes"— Levis, a T-shirt, and cowboy boots—and walked up the hill to the field. By the time I got there it was late in the game and the Ketchikan team was getting beaten soundly by the USS *Tortuga* team. My recollection was the score was something like 9–2, a high score for a fast-pitch softball game. In the top of the sixth inning, the *Tortuga* team scored twice more on the very tired Ketchikan pitcher.

During the bottom of the sixth when the Ketchikan team was getting ready to bat, I stepped out of the bleachers and walked over to the fence to talk to the guy who looked like he might have been the captain or manager of the home team. I told him I was a pitcher and if any teams in Ketchikan needed a pitcher I'd be in town for a while. He looked at me like I was an angel who had magically appeared before him and said, "*We* need a pitcher and we need one *now*. Our guy is dying out there and he doesn't think he can pitch one more inning. Can you finish the last inning for us?" My reaction was an incredulous laugh. "Naw, I can't do that. I've got cowboy boots on. I don't have my glove, and I'm not warmed up." "No problem," he said. "We'll find a glove and shoes that you can use and you've probably got five or ten minutes to warm up before we go out for the last inning." (Softball games are seven innings, not nine like baseball).

I thought for a brief moment about where I thought my blood sugar was. Of course, I didn't know for sure because self-testing was not possible then but I had eaten a big breakfast a couple of hours before and was pretty sure I'd be OK.

Well, he did get a left-handed glove for me but he couldn't find any size 14 shoes so I hopped over the fence in my cowboy boots and started warming up with their catcher. I threw only a dozen or so pitches before the Ketchikan team made their third out. As I walked out to the mound in my cowboy boots, I smiled to myself and thought that this was what guys dreamed about. They sit in the stands watching a game and say to themselves, "If I were out there, I could do better." Well, I was going to find out.

As I started taking my warm-up pitches from the mound, the radio announcer yelled down to the ump, "Who's the new pitcher?" The ump yelled to me from behind the plate, "What's your name?" "Mystrom," I shouted back. He then yelled up to the announcer, "Weisner." Well, I had more pressing things to think about than correcting my name with the radio announcer. After my three warm-up pitches, the game resumed.

Despite the fact that I walked the first guy after a 3-2 count, I could feel the buzz from the crowd because I was throwing so hard. Then I got into my groove and struck out the next three batters in a row. As I walked into the dugout, the guys were pretty excited—about as excited as a team can get when they're behind 11-2. The manager announced that I was fourth up so I might not get to bat. That was okay with me since I wasn't too sure about running bases in cowboy boots. But with two outs the batter in front of me got on base with a clean hit up the middle so I came up to bat. After watching two pitches, one ball and one strike, I hit the third one over the right field fence for a two-run homer. Good thing because I only had to trot around the bases.

It wasn't a game changer. I think the final score was 11-4 but the circumstances got a lot of attention. After hanging around the ballpark talking to players on both teams and a good number of curious spectators who wanted to know where I came from, I headed back to the hotel.

When I got back, Ricardo was still there reading and listening to the radio. As I walked in, he asked me where I had been. I told him I had been up at the game. As soon as I said that he sat up on the bed and asked if I had seen that guy "Weisner" who came out of the stands, struck out three guys and hit a home run. I said, "Yeh, that's me. I'm Weisner." Naturally, my name became Weisner for a while with our crew, and the radio station loved the story. For two days they led their sports news with "Spectator fans three and homers."

I never did play anymore in Ketchikan. Five days later, I was sent up to Juneau to help a crew up there. Another good break for me because that was Kathy Jeleski's hometown.

How Big Are You?

The work in Juneau was similar to that in Ketchikan, cutting sight lines for a road to be built north of Juneau. Lots of walking, cutting trees, and chopping down devil's club--an appropriately named noxious and prickly chest-high weed—with machetes.

I kept the same shot routine I had used in Ketchikan: a 10-unit shot of regular, fast-acting insulin in the morning followed by a large breakfast, then four hours of hard work and no shot for lunch. It seemed to work well but without testing, I really didn't know. I only knew that I was avoiding low blood sugar reactions and that was my priority.

The lessons I had learned from Ketchikan were clear: don't take long-lasting insulin on my days off, since the shot will carry over and impact the next day. And always have some sweets in my pocket for an emergency. I carried something sweet from that time on when I was out in the woods. I started with candy bars in my pocket but they, of course, melted and got a little messy. I switched to M&M's for a while but was too temped to eat them just because they tasted good. Then I switched to glucose tablets and finally, years later, to Skittles.

The only problem I had in Juneau was that I had filled out my paperwork for the job there. In the eyes of the federal government, Juneau was my home. Not a big deal except that it meant that I wouldn't get the 35-dollars-a-day per diem that I got in Ketchikan. It quickly became apparent that I would need to get a second job if I wanted to save any money.

I found an ad in the paper for a night clerk at the Northlander Hotel. I called the phone number in the ad and got a guy named Jim whose last name I can't seem to conjure up. I was expecting he would set an interview so he could meet me before he made a decision. But that wasn't necessary. After a little bit of small talk on the phone, he asked me the make-it-or-break-it-question. "How big are you?" When I told him I was 6 feet, 3 inches and about 215 pounds, he said with just a little hesitation, "That'll do. Meet me in the lobby at 8 p.m."

As we talked in the lobby, he explained that the job description was pretty simple. Protect the guests. Protect the property. And keep the peace. He explained that keeping the peace would be the biggest challenge since between about 2 a.m. and 4 a.m. all the bar patrons would spill onto the streets and bring their disagreements with them. Since the hotel was right next to the Red Dog Saloon, we would have action almost every night. Boy, was he right.

The sidewalks of downtown Juneau in 1968 between 2 and 4 a.m. were a cross between an English soccer riot and a Mike Tyson fight. Some fights went on for minutes, others were over in a matter of seconds. I generally didn't intervene unless the fight moved into the hotel lobby or unless someone in front of the hotel was clearly getting the worst of it. Then I'd jump in and usually, but not always, succeed in stopping it without becoming a combatant myself.

Because I kept with my routine of one shot of regular insulin before breakfast and one shot before dinner, I never had problems with low blood sugar during my nightly hotel adventures. Good thing, because one night all hell broke loose.

One morning about three o'clock, a bunch of pretty drunk patrons of the Red Dog stumbled out on the sidewalk right in front of the hotel ready to fight. From behind the hotel counter, I watched as at least three fights started outside the hotel. I hadn't decided whether or not to jump in when two of the drunks came fighting and sprawling into the hotel lobby. I jumped over the counter and dove into the middle of them. As I hit the fighters with my full weight, the cluster of the three of us moved toward the top of the stairs leading down to a Chinese restaurant on one side of the basement and the furnace room on the other. In a matter of seconds, we all started tumbling down the stairs. As soon as we hit bottom, I smelled smoke.

Nothing strikes fear into the heart of even the most novice hotelier as smoke in an old, wooden hotel with 50 guests asleep upstairs. This old wooden building also happened to be attached to every other old wooden building on the east side of Juneau's Franklin Street. I stepped over the back of one of the drunks, who had stopped fighting almost as if they understood something much more serious was happening. I opened the furnace room door and with the back draft of oxygen I let in, flames roared out the furnace room door.

I sprinted upstairs with singed hair and a bloody T-shirt and dialed "0" for an operator. She called the Juneau Volunteer Fire Department directly. Within seconds I heard the downtown horns give three short bursts over and over. That, to the best of my memory, was the signal for a fire downtown. With all the old, connected wooden structures in Juneau's town center, it wasn't hard for me to visualize the whole downtown burnt to the ground by sunrise and me trying to explain to the press why Alaska's capital city wasn't there anymore.

I slammed the receiver down and dashed up the stairs to start pounding on doors. That was our fire alarm system for the hotel. On the way up I met a shirtless, slightly overweight guest coming down to see what the commotion was. I told him to start beating on doors on the second floor. I took the third floor myself.

Three things stand out in my memory of that night. The first is how fast everyone woke up and ran out into the street in various stages of dress and undress. My second memory is the quick response of the volunteers of the fire department who held the fire to the furnace room and the stairwell. My third and most visual memory is standing on the street outside wearing a bloody shirt from breaking up the fight and trying to assure the owner—who had heard blasts from the siren and headed downtown to see if the fire was near his hotel—that everything was under control and he could go back to sleep. The Northlander hotel survived that night and is now called the Alaskan Hotel. Downtown Juneau survived that night and is still called Alaska's capital city.

Yakutat, Alaska

I was in the Juneau area for another month before I was sent up to Yakutat, a village of fewer than 500 people sitting hard on the Gulf of Alaska. My job was to help a crew up there survey a road being built from Yakutat to the Dangerous River. (I kid you not. That's really the name of the river.)

I lived in a big construction camp about 12 miles out of town. The camp consisted of basic portable wooden sleeping structures with bunk beds, shelves, and a cookshack that seated about 50 camp workers (eight surveyors and about 40 or so construction workers and heavy equipment operators). We were up at six every morning for breakfast and put in very physical days of walking, climbing, slashing brush, and cutting trees, and we often had some kind of physical competition in the evenings, mostly wrestling, footraces, relays, and football games.

We had only one day off, Sundays. Usually the survey crew, mostly college kids or recent graduates, went down to the beach and staged wrestling tournaments. I was one of the strongest guys but had never wrestled competitively and usually got beat by the smaller, weaker, but clearly more experienced college wrestlers among our crew.

After a couple of weeks in the construction camp, I was sorely missing female companionship. Unexpectedly, one day a letter reached me addressed to Rick Mystrom, general delivery, Yakutat, Alaska. It was from Kathy, the Alaska Airlines stewardess I had dated in Juneau. She said she had arranged to be in Yakutat overnight on a Sunday later that month and, "Could we get together?" Well, of course we could. It would be only a 12-mile Sunday morning stroll through the woods from camp to the town of Yakutat. Then I could easily get up at 3 a.m. Monday morning and walk back in time for a 6 a.m. breakfast before I started my day of hiking, brush-cutting, and surveying.

So that Sunday I hiked 12 miles through the woods to spend time with Kathy in Yakutat. Yakutat didn't offer a lot of social life, which was, of course, just fine with us. The challenge was to get up at 3 a.m. to walk the 12 miles back to the construction camp before the crew left in the back of a pickup truck to the work site for the day. But I didn't make it. Not only did I miss breakfast but I also missed the pickup truck that took the crew 5 miles to the work site for the day. So it turned out that I walked 17 miles just to start my workday. Amazing the impact young love has on a young man.

While working in Yakutat, I followed my same shot pattern: 10 units of regular insulin before a big breakfast, no shot at lunch and about 10 units before a big dinner. I didn't have any other low blood sugar episodes that summer. Looking back on this with what I've learned from testing my blood sugar levels over the past 30 years, I now realize why I had only one low blood sugar episode all that summer. My blood sugar was probably always high, though I had no way of knowing that at the time. I'm convinced that my very active and highly aerobic lifestyle helped maintain my health despite what I believe were almost 16 years of relatively high blood sugars before self-testing became available.

Leaving Alaska (at Least for a Few Years)

I finished my seasonal surveying job in early October and decided I couldn't leave Alaska without seeing the two biggest cities, Anchorage and Fairbanks. I flew up to Anchorage first and got together with some people I had met earlier that summer. It happened to be the weekend of Oktoberfest, a great party held in an old Quonset hut on Fireweed Lane, a street that was on the south edge of the city then. What went through my mind during that weekend was, "I like this city." What didn't enter my mind was that someday I would be the mayor of Anchorage.

Later that week I took the Alaska Railroad up to Fairbanks to spend a couple of days with Kathy, who had left Alaska Airlines to finish college at the University of Alaska in Fairbanks. By the time I left Alaska, I felt that someday I'd return.

You can give to your children just two things; the first is roots, the second is wings.

—Rick Mystrom (circa 1979)

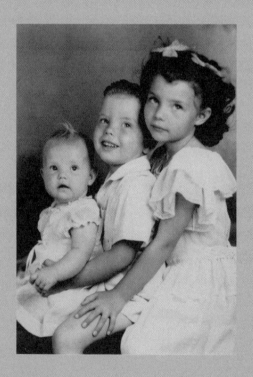

My little sister, Rochelle, was born October 9, 1946. As my sister, Rosanne, said in her book *Growing up Mystrom*, "This happy little girl completed our family."

Chapter 4

Growing Up Mystrom

After leaving Alaska, I headed back to Boulder, Colorado, where I could find friends who had an extra sofa or bed. Extra beds were a rarity but sofas were plentiful. I "crashed"—a '60s' term for sleeping on someone's sofa or floor—with my friend Art Horn, and within days I found a car, a four-year-old VW Beetle for $1,200, which turned out to be the start of my love affair with Volkswagens. Paying all cash would have left me with only about $200 and no job so I put $800 down and found a banker to loan me the $400 balance over two years. He must have counted my smile as collateral because that's all I had except for my books, four or five pairs of pants, a half dozen shirts, two pairs of shoes and one pair of boots and one jacket plus the suitcase that my mom and dad had given me for graduation.

Now I could get to Denver to begin looking for a job. Within a week I had two good job prospects, one with Texaco, whose recruiter offered me the job after the first interview then rejected me on the following day when I told him that I had diabetes. He told me that I would never pass their company physical. The other job prospect was with Uniroyal Tire Company in Joliet, Illinois. They weren't bothered by my diabetes.

They made me an offer as an industrial relations specialist. The recruiter said I'd be teaching classes to first-line supervisors in motivation, productivity, and communications. I accepted, put everything I owned in my VW and drove to Joliet.

My Dad and Mom

By the summer of 1969, I had been working at Uniroyal for less than a year when, at the age of 53, my dad had his second heart attack. He had always been a big, strong guy and a good dad. But I was always a little bit afraid of him. His most memorable threat to me was, "I'll kick your ass until your nose bleeds"—if I wore my pants too low, joked about my grandpa's Swedish accent, or got brought home by the cops. He actually never carried out that threat but it was a heck of a descriptive deterrent.

He had the demeanor of a charismatic tough guy but he loved us kids and never laid a hand on my sisters or my mom and not very often on me. He was a guard and correctional officer at some of the toughest prisons in the country: Stillwater and Sandstone, Minnesota; Lewisburg, Pennsylvania; Inglewood, Colorado; and Terminal Island in California. More than once I heard him referred to by other guards as the toughest of the guards. I never actually cranked up enough courage to ask him how he got that reputation.

But to my sisters and me, he wasn't the toughest of the guards. He was just "dad"—fun, caring, well-spoken, and athletic. He had an excellent command of the English language and expected, but never demanded, the same from us kids. I always admired his easy and graceful athleticism. He was good at whatever sports were in season and never seemed to have to work hard at them. He had a natural coordination and smoothness that combined to make him look graceful at whatever he did. To this day I can visualize how he glided gracefully around the frozen lakes on his prewar speed skates. And in the summer I would watch in awe as he swam faster and more smoothly than all the other dads while wearing his old blue woolen swimsuit with a knit belt and metal buckle.

My dad had been in the U.S. Navy during World War II. His ship, *LST 379*, had landed at Salerno and Anzio in Italy and at Normandy on June 6, 1944 as part of the invasion of Nazi-occupied France. That invasion led to the death of Hitler, the freeing of Europe from Nazi Germany, and the

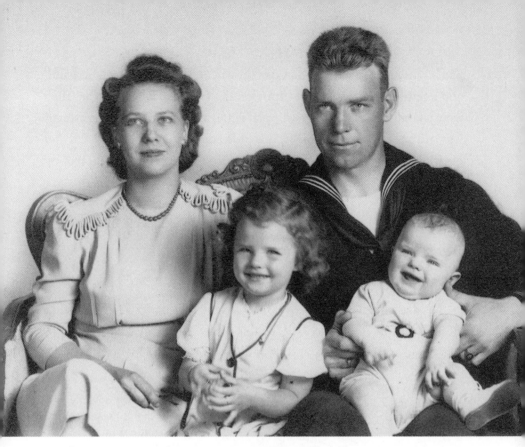

Our family, not long before the invasion at Normandy.

My mom and dad, my big sister, Rosanne, and me, the little chubby guy. Rochelle, my younger sister, was not yet born.

liberation of surviving prisoners from the horrific Nazi death camps. After victory in Europe (VE Day), his ship set sail through the Panama Canal to Leyte Bay in the Philippines to prepare for the invasion of Japan. That invasion, of course, never happened. Emperor Hirohito announced Japan's surrender on August 15, 1945.

My first vague memory of my dad was in our backyard in Sandstone, Minnesota a couple of years after he was discharged from the U.S. Navy. I was either three or four years old. Dad and some friends were standing around his old black 1936 Ford parked on our back lawn near the alley. He had his foot on the running board of the car, a Camel cigarette in his hand, and a bottle of Hamm's beer sitting on the front fender of the car. They were talking about how they whipped Hitler and Tojo (Japan's minister of war and later prime minister). I was little and I thought that my dad and his friends were so big of course they won. I couldn't imagine anybody whipping them.

Chrissy Thorvig, Susie Davis, and I imitated our dads at war by playing war games. We'd run around our yard, arms outstretched like airplanes, a rock in each pudgy little four-year-old fist and when we passed our sandbox filled with army men and army trucks we'd drop our rocks and yell out, "Bombs over Tokyo!"

My dad got a letter after the war from the Secretary of the Navy that clearly and concisely described the role of the American sailors in World War II and expressed the gratitude of their country. The letter read, in part:

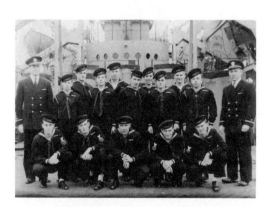

Left: The bridge crew of *LST 379.* My dad is the tall one, standing fifth from the left. He was the ship's radar man.

Bottom: My dad's ship on the beach at Normandy. Probably about D-Day plus 3.

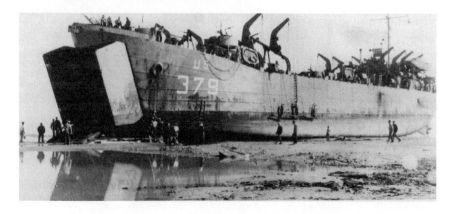

January 26, 1946

My dear Mr. Mystrom:

... You have served in the greatest navy in the world. It
has crushed two enemy fleets at once, receiving their
surrenders only four months apart. It brought our land-
based air power within bombing range of the enemy,
and set our armies on the beachheads of final victory.
No other navy at any time has done so much. For your
part in these achievements you deserve to be proud for
as long as you live. The nation which you served at a
time of crisis will remember you with gratitude.

James Forrestal
Secretary of the Navy

I flew back home to Garden Grove, California when my dad first went
into the hospital with his second heart attack. After a few days, he seemed
to be getting stronger so my mom and my sisters suggested it would be
okay for me to fly back to Illinois.

I stopped by the hospital to see my dad on my way to the airport. We
talked casually about how he was feeling, about my job, about the girl I was
dating, and about the softball team I was pitching for. As I left my dad's
hospital room to head to the airport, we were both sure we'd see each other
again and as I turned around to wave goodbye, he put his right hand to his
forehead in a casual salute—which was his way of saying goodbye—a habit
he'd had since his navy days. He raised his head, smiled at me, and said,
"Let me know if you need a good third baseman." Those were the last words
he ever said to me.

Two days after I got back to Joliet, my sister, Rosanne, called me with
two other words I'll never forget: "Daddy died."

My doctors have periodically expressed concern about his early death
and a genetic predisposition I might have to the same short life span. But

for my dad it was probably caused by the two packs of Camels he smoked every day for most of his life combined with not much exercise and a traditional '40s' and '50s' diet of meat, mashed potatoes and gravy almost every day. Fortunately, I've never smoked except for an occasional cigar and I've always been very physically active. Because of diabetes, I've learned what and when to eat in order to live a healthy and long life. I now honestly believe that I will live longer because of what I've learned about food and health than I would have had I not had diabetes.

We were always a small family. Both my parents were only children so my two sisters and I had no uncles or aunts or first cousins. Now we were smaller by one. My mom continued to care for her father—Grandpa Herman to us kids—who had been living with her and my dad for about five years. He had emigrated from Sweden during the potato famine in northern Europe at the turn of the century and worked in logging camps in northern Minnesota for years to save enough money to bring his brothers and sisters to America. After a career as a successful home builder in St. Paul, Minnesota, he lost everything he had in the Great Depression. He continued working as a carpenter before retiring to manage an apartment building until his wife, Ella, died. Then he moved to California to live with my mom and dad. Grandpa Herman was a true hero of our family. He worked hard and earned a good living for his family back in the days when self-earned success was a virtue.

My first clear memory of Mom was when I was four years old in Sandstone, Minnesota. I can't quite conjure up what I had done to make her mad. It was something I did in the front yard of our little house. She came walking quickly and firmly out of the house toward me with a stern look on her face. When she got so close that I knew it wasn't a bluff charge, I ran down the sidewalk in front of our house. I knew I was faster than my friends, Susie Davis and Chrissy Thorvig, but I didn't know if I was faster than Mom. It turned out that I was. As I turned around to see if she was catching me, I saw her stop and take off one of her brown loafers. She threw it at me as I continued running as fast as my four-year-old legs could go when the shoe hit me square in the back of the head. It knocked me—as my dad would say "ass over teakettle"—onto the sidewalk screaming with

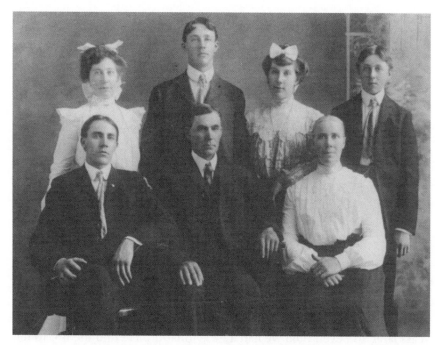

Grandpa Herman (Herman Elmer, center, standing) was the hero of our family. He held his family together and led them all toward positive lives after their mother died and their father (seated) committed suicide in jail.

skinned knees. Mom immediately shifted from "mad mom" to "caring mom" and brought me into the kitchen where she did all the bandaging of us kids.

It was the only time I can recall that she did anything that hurt me physically. She infused my sisters and me with love and caring all our lives and never wavered in her support for us.

Lewisburg, Pennsylvania

We moved to Lewisburg, Pennsylvania in 1949 when I was five. My dad had been transferred from the federal prison in Sandstone, Minnesota to the maximum-security Lewisburg penitentiary—sort of an eastern US version of Alcatraz. We lived in one-half of a small duplex at 334 North Fourth Street, which my mom and dad rented for 35 dollars a month. Mom furnished it neatly and kept it clean and comfortable. She was a wonderful role model, a strong defender of my sisters and me, a gracious hostess, and a habitual party-line enforcer— "… Mrs. Howard, get off the party line. I know you're listening." She was a wonderful cook but often a day or two before payday when the "icebox" was empty, we had fried oatmeal patties with sugar and butter, which my sisters and I viewed as a treat, not a hardship. In those days credit cards did not exist. When we were out of money, we waited until my dad's next paycheck.

Although we never had much money, my sisters and I never thought of ourselves as poor. It didn't enter our minds to be envious of our friends who lived in nicer homes or whose parents even owned their home. After all, we had bikes. Mom and Dad saved to buy Rosanne and me a Hawthorne bike from Montgomery Ward's on our eighth birthdays. My dad confided in me that mine had cost almost 11 dollars, which was two dollars more than Rosanne's bike. Of course, my eighth birthday was more than two years later and even then we had a little inflation. He told me not to tell her. I never did—until now. By the time it was my little sister Rochelle's turn to get her bike, the money was tighter so my dad fixed up Rosanne's blue and gray six-year-old Hawthorne bike and gave it to Rochelle on her eighth birthday.

Lewisburg provided my sisters and me a wonderful small-town American childhood. My friends and I spent our summers riding bikes all over town and often into the countryside for miles. My favorite riding area was the Bucknell University campus because of the hills and asphalt footpaths that provided our version of a roller coaster that could get us up to 30 miles per hour according to Mark Betzer's bike speedometer.

Our favorite adventure hike was a couple of miles out of town along the Susquehanna River to an area we called Red Rocks. We hiked all over the area and often came home with Indian arrowheads, boyhood treasures I still have. My sisters and I became best friends as we played together, laughed together, and adventured together.

My sister Rosanne describes our childhood beautifully in a book she produced for our family titled *Growing Up Mystrom: Memories of the 1940s and '50s*.

There was always plenty of activity around the Mystrom household with us three kids and lots of friends who gathered at our house in Pennsylvania or wherever we lived to play hide and seek, ride our bikes along country roads in the summertime, or go sledding on Meter's hill—just a block away—during the winter months.

Mother was a great cook and there were always cookies for friends and sumptuous meals for relatives who came to stay.

It was a wonderful childhood.

Baseball, bicycles, and slingshots seemed to be a big part of my memories of Lewisburg. I started playing Little League baseball at the age of eight. I was the only eight-year-old on a team of mostly 10-, 11-, and 12-year-olds. I wasn't as strong or fast as the older kids but I could catch pretty well. I remember my coach telling me "Richie, I'm going to put you in right field. You're not as fast as the older kids but if the ball comes close to you, you'll catch it."

Fifty-two years later I was 60 years old and still playing softball in a competitive league in Anchorage. My coach was my longtime friend, Rod Hill. After about the third game of the year, Rod pulled me aside and said, "Rick, I'm going to put you in right field. You're not as fast as the younger guys but if the ball comes close to you, you'll catch it." I had heard that more than a half century before. Four years later at 64 and after 56 years of playing baseball or softball, I stopped playing. But I couldn't stay away from that wonderful American game. I started playing again last summer at 68, for a 50-and-older team.

When we were kids, honesty and family support were drilled into us. I got into trouble once when I lied to my parents about a fight I had been in. My eye was almost swollen shut. So I told them what most 10-year-old boys would tell their parents. "I was playing baseball and a grounder took a bad hop and hit me in the eye." It was a pretty good shiner and my eye was almost swollen closed, so Mom said I didn't have to go to school that morning. As

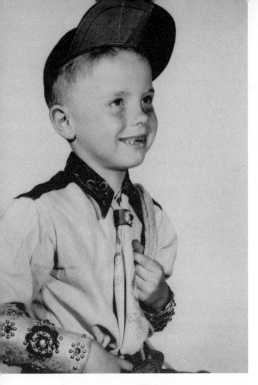

At seven years old I was unsure about whether I wanted to be a cowboy or a baseball player.

I was lying in bed gloating about all the *Hopalong Cassidy, Lash Larue,* and *Captain Marvel* comic books I could read that day, even with one eye, I heard Rochelle's girlfriend, Jeannie Lockwood, who came to our house every morning to walk to school with my sister, say to my dad, "You should have seen the fight Richie was in yesterday." Well, that was the end of my day off. The toughest prison guard wasn't going to let his son stay home from school because of a black eye he got in a fight. I had to cut the grass for a couple of weeks and dig a stump out of our backyard for that lie.

The honesty message was fresh in my mind later that summer when I told my 12-year-old big sister, Rosanne, I could throw a rock farther than she could shoot a rock with my slingshot. I suggested that we stand at the corner of our alley and Beck Street and throw toward Fourth Street. She agreed. Rosanne went first and shot a rock with my slingshot farther than I thought she could. I knew I'd need to give my throw everything I had. I put my full 70 pounds behind a monster throw. But as soon as it left my hand I knew it was off target. It was going straight toward the house on the corner of the street where Marshall Mark Blank lived alone. I don't know what kind of a marshal he was but all of us kids were afraid to talk to him. We presumed he never got married because he was too scary.

The moment the rock headed toward his house, I sensed trouble and stepped behind the garage into the alley. Then I heard the breaking of glass, the instantaneous opening of a door and the booming voice of Marshall Blank yelling, "Who the hell did that?" There in the middle of the street with a slingshot dangling from her hand and a bewildered look on her face stood Rosanne.

As she stood there, he started walking toward her. In one of the prouder moments in my young life and with the memory of my previous lie still fresh, I stepped out from behind the garage and said, "I did it."

That worked out pretty well for me. I got a lot of credit for being honest and no criticism for hiding behind the garage in the first place and leaving my sister standing out there alone with the slingshot in her hand.

Working for the federal government, my dad got two weeks of vacation every year. So each year for all five years we lived in Lewisburg our vacations were the same—a two-week stay in Minnesota to visit relatives. It was about a 1,200-mile trip according to my dad, and we could afford only one stay in a motel room at seven dollars a night. With no four-lane highways, every road we took meant stop-and-starting through towns and not around them, so we had two long days in the car.

The night before we left mom always packed our suitcase and made sandwiches, Dad loaded our 1949 Studebaker Commander, and each of us kids had three comic books we bought at Newberry's five-and-ten-cent store. Rosanne, Rochelle, and I were always so excited we couldn't sleep. We knew what was coming. The next morning Mom would be in to wake us up at 3:30 a.m. The excitement of being awake and sneaking around quietly when the rest of Lewisburg was asleep brought some sort of odd excitement to our departure.

The vacations themselves—visiting our mom's and dad's cousins, playing with new friends, going to the Como Park Zoo, spending a few days on our relative's farm, fishing with Grandpa Dick—left wonderful and enduring memories. Mary and I have worked consciously to give our children vacation experiences that I hope will find that same special place in their childhood memories.

In Lewisburg I also had my first girlfriend, Sherry Zechman, who was about 6 inches taller than I and pretty gangly. But she was a fast runner and very smart. That's important in the sixth grade. She was also the May Queen of South Ward Elementary and I was only on the May Court, not the May King, so I didn't really have first dibs on Sherry. But she was my girlfriend anyway, which meant that she wore my jacket and held hands with me after school. On our first date, I took her to a matinee at the Campus theatre and spent the biggest part of the movie working my right arm over the back of her seat and down onto her shoulders. I figured at that rate of progress, it would take me at least six months to work up to a kiss. But before that happened, my dad got transferred to Terminal Island, a federal prison in Long Beach, California, and I never did kiss Sherry.

Garden Grove, California

When we first moved to California, my parents bought one of the thousands of small tract houses being built in Orange County in the '50s. Our house was in Garden Grove, an unincorporated community of about 15,000 people in Orange County. The advertised price for a house in our tract was "less than $10,000" and the final papers showed my folks bought it for $9,999. 99

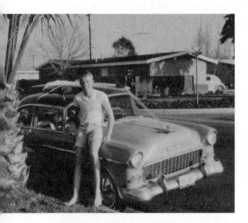

One of the last photos taken of me before being diagnosed with diabetes. Note how thin I was there. Not long after I started taking insulin, I developed, in the words of Dr. Daarud, "a much more powerful physique." Insulin doesn't, by itself, create an athletic physique but it does provide the opportunity for both young men and women to build healthy, athletic physiques.

As an aside I used to entertain my nephews and neighborhood kids by vaulting over that car (without the surfboard) and landing in the street. It still amazes me that I did that stunt barefoot.

It would be three months before the house would be finished so we rented a small apartment in Long Beach about 12 blocks from the Pike Amusement Park on the waterfront. Rosanne was 14, I was 11, and Rochelle was 9. Since we had no other friends, my sisters and I spent the summer hanging out together at the beach and at the Pike on Wednesdays when all the park rides were 10 cents.

My sisters and I have been lifelong friends. Playmates when we were young, confidantes as we got older, and supporters and mentors as adults. They both have wonderful and successful husbands and families as well as a history of success in their own careers. My dad would have been proud of all their accomplishments. My mom was.

Meeting Mary

It was at Dad's funeral that I first saw Mary, a beautiful, brown-eyed, tanned California girl by way of Wisconsin. I asked my sister Rochelle who she was. She told me that she was going to school at a nearby college and managing the bakery at the local supermarket. Rochelle said that Dad always stopped to talk (and probably flirt) with her whenever he was in the store. I later found out that he had told Mary that "my son and I don't agree on a lot of things but I'm pretty sure that we'd agree on you." As it turned out, he was right. Some family friends arranged for me to go on a date with her before I went back to Joliet. We went to the Garden Grove Strawberry Festival. I won her a big stuffed turtle and she won my heart. She was beautiful, smart, and fun.

Two weeks later, I resigned from Uniroyal, and once again, packed everything I owned in my VW and headed from Illinois to California. My head said it was to help my mom, but my heart said it was to see Mary.

The Similar Symptoms of Heat Stroke and Extreme Low Blood Sugar

I didn't exactly walk over hot coals to see Mary again but I came pretty close. When I got to the Arizona–California border on my way to Garden Grove, it was 126 degrees. The border officials were recommending everyone turn around and go back to Kingman, Arizona or wait until sundown to drive the 100 or so miles across the Mojave Desert to Needles, the nearest town in California. But I was on a mission and turning back wasn't part of it. I ignored their advice and went on.

My 1964 VW had no air conditioning and worse yet, the back windows didn't roll down. When I rolled down the front windows, I got blasted with 126-degree air at 70 miles per hour. So I kept rolling the windows down and back up. Both situations were pretty much intolerable. If it was 126 outside it must have been 20 degrees hotter inside that little oven of a car.

Somewhere around the point of no return, about 50 miles out, I realized I had not seen another car since I left the border. About that same time blinding white flashes started lighting up my head—about 10 minutes apart at first then closer as the miles crept by. My options weren't good. In fact, I had no options: no shade, no water, and no other cars.

I willed myself to stay conscious. The flashes seemed to be only a few minutes apart. In the distance, I saw a bowling alley on the outskirts of Needles. Getting there was like a slow-motion dream—the car was moving but it didn't seem to get any closer. After an eternity I reached the life-saving bowling alley.

Getting out of the car and walking into the building was pure focus and willpower. "Stay on your feet," I kept telling myself. "Keep your eyes on the door. You'll make it." But I couldn't put together thoughts in any linear fashion. I was lurching forward in bright, flashing staccato steps. My eyes were fixed on the door. I willed myself forward.

And finally I made it to the bowling alley door. Inside some patrons started bringing me glasses of water, which I alternated drinking and pouring over my head. I spent over an hour in that air-conditioned building before I felt good enough to keep going.

Years later, after having a number of low blood sugar reactions, I came to realize that my symptoms of impending heatstroke that day were almost identical to the symptoms of severe low blood sugar: a sense of brightness, confusion, lack of linear thinking, inability to put thoughts together, and finally, before you pass out, flashes of light. I remember waking up many times, before I learned how to better control my nighttime blood sugar level, in the middle of the night with very low blood sugar and the same kind of brightness and lights flashing in my head. It would take the same kind of narrow focus for me to work my way downstairs to the refrigerator, only to stand there with the door open with the needed orange juice or soft drink right in front of me, but often uncertain about what to do.

I lived at my mom's house for a while, helping her adjust to my dad's death, then got a job at Mattel Toys and moved to an apartment in Manhattan Beach. Life was good. Mary and I had started dating regularly. I liked my job and the people I was working with and was soon competing on Mattel's football, basketball, and fast-pitch softball teams in the highly competitive Southern California leagues.

Mattel was loaded with bright, creative, and interesting people. Derek Gable, a toy designer, was the most creative person I've ever known and to this day is a close friend. Herschel Kranitz, whom I've lost touch with, was a smart, funny, lovable, and fascinating guy who still causes people to light up 40 years later whenever his name comes up in conversation. Watching and learning from two other bright Mattel employees, Joe Zacarro and Don Payne, helped prepare me for running my own businesses years later.

My First Extreme Low Blood Sugar Reaction

One of my best friends at Mattel was Bill Keenan, whom I knew from my days in Joliet. He was an aggressive go-getter I recommended to Mattel's top recruiter as a great prospect for the company. He was subsequently hired by Mattel and moved to Southern California about six months after I did. Shortly after Bill arrived at Mattel, I suggested that we go to Las Vegas for the weekend. To a guy like Bill who'd seen only Joliet, Chicago, and LA, going to Las Vegas was, in Mattel jargon, like real-life Barbie dolls and Hot Wheels. He was ready.

It was on this trip that I had my first *extreme* low blood sugar reaction resulting in a seizure and an ambulance trip to the emergency room. It's the only extreme reaction that I don't remember with clarity, either the circumstances or the specific error I made that caused the incident. Once I had my first two extreme reactions, I became much more attuned to the cause and effect and could identify specifically what "pilot error" caused each episode.

Our second night in Las Vegas was a typical night of fun, laughter, and low-stakes gambling. Bill and I had been drinking, not heavily, but pretty consistently, throughout the night (a pattern I fortunately grew out of pretty early in my adult life). I recall drinking rum and Cokes. We got back to our hotel room about two or three in the morning. I guessed that my blood sugar was probably high because of the Coke in the drinks. I gave myself an additional shot of insulin and then quickly fell asleep (of course this was 1969, still way before self-testing of blood sugar).

The next thing I remember is a vague conversation of people around me in white smocks. I heard the words "diabetic," "insulin shock," and "… looks like he's coming around." As my life came back into focus, I realized I was in a hospital. I remembered who I was but not what happened. I asked the attending doctor. According to him, I had suffered a seizure around

4 a.m. and Bill had called an ambulance. Bill told me later that I fought with the ambulance attendants and it took both attendants and Bill to get me strapped to a gurney.

It was my first seizure requiring emergency help. I felt okay except for a black eye I got from falling face first onto the floor. The doctor said it looked like I was going to be fine and he would release me in a couple of hours.

I was out of the Las Vegas hospital by midmorning and Bill and I headed back to LA. Since this was before the days that I was open about my diabetes, I asked him not to say anything about what happened. With my black eye that wasn't easy for Bill or me but sometimes silence can create mystery.

This was my first extreme reaction and I didn't yet understand that it could happen repeatedly unless I developed an in-depth understanding of the relationship between food, insulin, and exercise. I have since learned that sequences preceding a seizure caused by an extreme low blood sugar reaction are the same: First, your memory blanks out even before you lose consciousness; second, you can move around a room, a house, or even a hotel and not be aware of it; and third, you don't feel anything, see anything, think anything, or even dream anything until you start to regain consciousness. Subsequent reactions followed this pattern. My first post-seizure memories would always be hearing the emergency room doctors or paramedics around me talking.

The recovery to consciousness is typically a result of the emergency medical technicians or the emergency room doctors inserting an IV with what's called DW50—50 percent dextrose and 50 percent water. It's like a huge sugar boost that brings you back quickly.

My Second Extreme Low Blood Sugar Reaction

In October 1970, Mary and I got married. After a fun, weeklong honeymoon to San Francisco and Lake Tahoe (first night at the Santa Barbara Biltmore and the rest at Howard Johnson's) we returned to our little house in Southcentral LA that we had rented for 85 dollars a month. It was actually in the backyard of another small house and looked more like a medium-sized travel trailer than a house. But Mary made curtains and drapes, put up wallpaper, planted flowers, and made it a warm, cozy home. It was our tiny piece of paradise among the roars of motorcycles, the wail of sirens, and the periodic gunshots that often woke us up at night.

In June 1971, I had my second extreme low blood sugar reaction requiring an emergency room trip. Bruce Burba was a partying friend of mine from my Joliet days. We had gone to both Mardi Gras and the Kentucky Derby together in the year after he had graduated from Northwestern and I from the University of Colorado. He had decided to come to California for some reason or for no reason. Bruce didn't need a reason to do anything. Just a little money in his pocket and a desire for fun was motivation enough.

He showed up, occupied our sofa for a few days —then a few more days—then a few more days. During his continuing stay we had invented some multiskilled competitions in our driveway involving footballs, basketballs, and softballs. I had given myself a normal shot of insulin for dinner which I later recalled was mostly roast beef. (This was my first lesson on how little protein will raise blood sugar.) After dinner we got into competitions which lasted a couple of hours.

By the time Mary and I settled into our bed and Bruce once again settled his over-6-foot frame onto our under-6-foot sofa, my blood sugar was probably low and going down. Since exercise increases the impact of insulin by further lowering blood sugar, it was as if I had taken a much larger dose of insulin. That exercise combined with a low- or no-carbohydrate meal was an extreme low blood sugar episode in the making. It's another illustration of the importance for all insulin-dependent diabetics to thoroughly understand the relationship between food, activity, and insulin.

What happened next could only be described in detail by Mary or Bruce. In short, my blood sugar got too low too fast. I started convulsing. Mary yelled for Bruce to help. Bruce held me down while Mary called an ambulance. The next thing I remember was waking up in the emergency room with people in white coats around me. As I started to come to, a nurse brought Mary in to help me gain my sense of place. She remembers my looking at her and saying, "Oh, you're pregnant." She was—about eight months' worth. Since it was late at night, they kept me in the hospital until the next morning. It was one of the few times I've been kept overnight for an extreme low blood sugar episode.

It was the second time within a year that I had to be taken to the hospital in an ambulance because my blood sugar got too low at night. Because of these two episodes and since I had no way to measure my blood sugar, I started focusing on being sure I ate something before I went to bed. Oftentimes that something was ice cream or sweets, which was not a good idea, but my goal above all else was to avoid another seizure.

After glucose self-testing became available a number of years later and I could measure my blood sugars myself, everything changed. From that point on, I would almost always be aware of what my blood sugar was before I went to bed. Being able to measure my blood sugars made me realize how high my blood sugar levels must have been in the premeasurement days. It also took away the need to eat sweets before I went to bed. I think I can say without doubt if glucose monitors had not been invented, I would not be alive today.

An interesting aside to that episode was that I found a doctor in the phone book and went to him for advice. His diagnosis was that I probably had epilepsy and he prescribed antiseizure medication, which I took for about six months before I finally surmised that his diagnosis was wrong.

Because my blood sugars were so high so often, I believe the only thing that kept me healthy was my year-round sports activity for Mattel's competitive teams. I played wide receiver on their football team, pitcher and left fielder on their softball team, forward on their basketball team, and even gave soccer and rugby a shot—soccer I wasn't very good at but I was judged by my Aussie friends as pretty good at rugby for a Yank.

A month after that low blood sugar episode and nine months to the day after we got married, our first child, Nicholas Roger, was born. Mary set up a cozy little crib area for Nicky in the hallway of our tiny house. Always very supportive of my sports activities she took Nicky on his first outing to one of my softball games when he was only five days old. I obviously was very inspired by his attendance because I pitched a no-hitter and went 4 for 4 at the plate with two home runs and two doubles. I've always kept the inscribed and signed ball given to me by the team that night. It's dated July 21, 1971.

Once You've Been to Alaska, You Never Go All the Way Home

I had been in Southern California for a little over three years and Mary and I had been married for about a year and a half but we never really connected to Southern California. I had talked about Alaska a lot with Mary and she knew that I'd like to move there someday and give it a shot. She was willing. After all, we had $750 in our savings account and a pretty reliable Volkswagen van. On the challenging side of the ledger, we had an eight-month-old baby and a dog, and it just happened to be February. But the lure of Alaska won out and I was becoming a believer that "once you've been to Alaska, you never go all the way home."

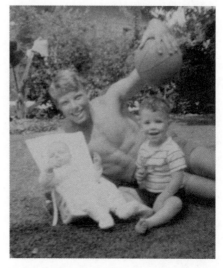

Two of my nephews, Ron and Steve Bader, and I just before Mary and I left for Alaska.

Nothing is given beneath the sun;

Nothing is had that is not won.

—Swedish Hymn

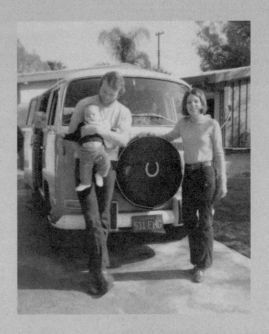

The day Mary and I left Southern California
for Alaska in a VW van with our eight-
month-old son, Nick, and our life
savings of $750.

Chapter 5

North to Alaska for Good
*In February, 1972 with $750 and
an Eight-Month-Old Baby*

Derek Gable and His Test

"You're crazy! What are you thinking about? Alaska? In the middle of winter?"

It was Derek being Derek. "I could understand it, Rick, if you were going up with a group of lads." Being from England, Derek never learned to speak "American." He still spoke English. Guys were "lads" and girls were "birds." Sausage and potatoes were "bangers and mash" and leftovers were "bubble and squeak." He was part of a clan of British inventors of toys at Mattel Toy Company, where I worked. They were almost all lads and definitely big contributors to Mattel's extraordinary success in the 1960s.

"I can't believe you're going to Alaska in a Volkswagen van, pulling an overweight, ugly, tongue-heavy, homemade blue plywood trailer," Derek exclaimed. "And you're taking your wife, an eight-month-old baby, and a dog. Unbelievable. Not to mention that you have no job and only $750 to your name. Plus you're leaving in the middle of winter!" To Derek's credit he never mentioned diabetes as a problem. And honestly, it never entered my mind as a reason to be apprehensive about our adventure. Derek just thought the only problem I had was a case of stupid.

I have to admit when he strung it all together like that it did seem pretty stupid. I think the only people in LA who thought we'd make it were the same people who thought the Dodgers were going to win the World Series the next year. So I quit asking friends for opinions. Problem solved.

Derek grumbled good-naturedly the whole time he helped me load the trailer with our sparse household belongings. When we got it loaded, the trailer design, or lack thereof, made it so tongue-heavy that it lifted the front wheels of my VW van off the ground. This confirmed in Derek's mind that my decision-making ability was somewhat south of a junior high dropout's. We unloaded and reloaded the trailer with all the heavy stuff as far back as possible.

When we were finally reloaded and the front wheels stayed down, Derek came up with a plan—as he always did. We'd pretest the trip by pulling the trailer up Palos Verdes hill, a pretty stiff 5-mile climb from the bottom to the top. Derek's proposal was if my VW van made it up the hill pulling that heavy trailer we'd have at least an outside chance of making it to Alaska. He figured that if we didn't make it up the hill and if the engine or transmission burned out, I'd have to get it fixed and wouldn't have any money left to go anyway. Derek said he'd ask the birds, our wives, if they wanted to go. They did. Mary, Pam, Derek, and I all piled in, intent on confirming our own preexisting opinions.

As we started up the hill, I knew it wasn't going to be a slam dunk. I had quickly downshifted to second but that wasn't enough. I had to downshift to low gear right away. VW vans have five-speed transmissions and low gear in a VW five-speed is *really* low—like 5 miles per hour low. It doesn't take much of a mathematician to realize that a 5-mile hill at 5 miles per hour is going to take you, well—about an hour. Plenty of time for Derek and me to argue about whether 5 miles an hour was really making it or not. I pointed out that we were passing the stragglers in some sort of an uphill race that was going on. He pointed out that it was a footrace, not a car race. My argument weakened when we got to the middle of the pack and were only holding our own while in the distance we could see the leaders pulling away from us.

We made it to the top. I declared victory even though the burning smell of the overheated engine hung heavy inside the van. Derek declared that by his calculation Mary and I would completely miss the winter in Alaska, which he thought was a good thing. He also surmised that we would likely miss spring and arrive midsummer and that at least the highway wouldn't be snow-packed.

The trip down the hill was much easier although the smell of burning brakes gave Derek's arguments new life. In a show of good sportsmanship Derek and Pam invited us over for the "Last Supper"—bubble and squeak, of course. We said our goodbyes to them and to our other friends and family.

Two days later Mary, eight-month-old Nicky, our dog, Tara, and I left for Alaska with a packed van and a full trailer. We towed the trailer as far as Tacoma, Washington, loaded it on a barge, and caught the Alaska Marine Highway ferry out of Vancouver to Haines, Alaska, which left us with a two-day midwinter drive on a narrow snow-packed road over Chilkat Pass to the Alaska Highway, then on to Anchorage.

Alaska's (Future) Most Famous Wildlife Photographer

Luckily we met Johnny Johnson on the ferry. That meeting on the ferry was the beginning of a lifelong friendship with Johnny and his wife, Kathy, who came up later that year. Johnny became Alaska's premier wildlife photographer and Kathy became a highly respected and honored schoolteacher. When Johnny and Kathy divorced many years later, she remarried another terrific guy, Rich Huffman. Kathy and Rich were tragically killed in June, 2005 by a barren-ground grizzly near the Brooks Range in Northern Alaska.

When we met Johnny on the ferry he was on his way to climb Mount McKinley and was loaded with cold-weather gear. He had one parka that was designed for something like 50 degrees below zero. He lent that to Mary so she could keep Nick wrapped up with her for the duration of the trip. We planned to caravan together along with a lady named Ethel who was going to Kenai, Alaska to find her "loser of a husband" as she referred to him, who had left her a couple of years before.

We spent the night in Haines and left in a three-vehicle caravan at daybreak the next morning. It was 20 degrees below zero with limited visibility and blowing snow. I soon discovered that trying to heat a VW van with its inadequate little heater is like trying to heat a hotel with a candle. It actually never got above freezing *inside* the van and we had to deal with frozen baby formula and frozen dog food until Mary put those provisions inside the parka too.

We left Haines early the next morning. Not only was it very cold but it was also overcast. We couldn't see much beyond a mile so the beautiful scenery Mary was anticipating was invisible. As we started to climb the Chilkat Pass, a 3,500-foot pass just north of Haines, the very first scene Mary saw in Alaska was a derelict tractor-trailer truck lying on its side and partially blocking the road. It looked very much like it had been there for months and probably wouldn't be removed until spring. To Mary's credit she still never exhibited any trepidation or hesitation about going forward.

After a couple of small incidents—not diabetes related—we made it to Anchorage two days later. Johnny headed north to prepare for his ascent of Mount McKinley. Mary and I rented a tiny apartment at 2702 Denali Street in Anchorage for about $150 a month, as I recall. Our remaining cash, before shopping for groceries, was less than $200 but we had a tax refund of $272 coming, which turned out to be what kept us going until I got my first paycheck about a month later.

Starting out in Anchorage

We had made it to Anchorage. Now I had to get a job—fast. The first day I applied for a job at Kinney's Shoes but didn't get it. I like to think that I was overqualified, but maybe not. That evening we were watching the news on our little 12-inch black and white TV set and I said to Mary, "There's an opportunity. Their regular newscaster must have just died and they've got someone off the street to fill in until they get a new one. I'll apply for the job as newscaster tomorrow."

Accidental Ad Man

The next day I walked into KIMO-TV, the ABC affiliate station in Anchorage. It was a small, two-story office building on the edge of town. The receptionist was an attractive, slightly pudgy lady who I soon found out was the wife of the company president. We seemed to hit it off well and after a few minutes of small talk, she excused herself to go to talk to the president (her husband). I don't know what she said to him but she came back and said he'd like to

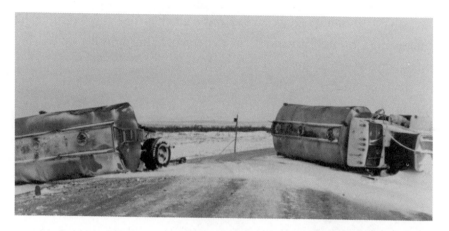

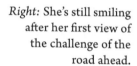

Top: Mary's introduction to Alaska scenery.

Right: She's still smiling after her first view of the challenge of the road ahead.

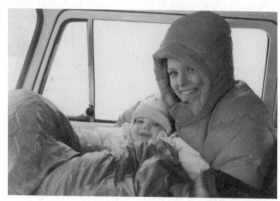

see me. I walked upstairs and into his office with no idea what skills being a TV newscaster required other than a low voice and a decent appearance.

I put on my deepest bass voice, which is deeper than Death Valley, and announced that I was just up from LA and was interested in doing his evening newscasts. Well I must have sounded like James Earl Jones with a cold, because the first question he asked me was, "Do you always talk like that?" That broke the ice. We both started laughing and I said, "Nope. I can talk normal too." After a short conversation, he asked me how much I needed to make. I hadn't really thought about that and the most that could come out of my mouth without swallowing hard was $1,000 a month. He told me that I couldn't make that kind of money starting out in the news but I could in advertising sales.

After a 30-minute conversation and a quick glance at my résumé, he offered me a job at $750 a month or 15 percent of my monthly advertising sales, whichever was greater. I accepted.

That began a career in advertising—a career that would span 22 years and lead to involvement with most of Alaska's political leaders, with the United States Olympic Committee (USOC), the International Olympic Committee (IOC), four American presidents, and a cluster of other world leaders. My advertising career would end when I sold my ad agency to run for mayor.

Nearly Drowning under a Logjam

We didn't have much money that summer but we did save enough to buy a used, 16-foot yellow fiberglass canoe for $75. It was in that canoe that I had my first near-death experience in Alaskan waters. Mary and I used the canoe primarily to go down Campbell Creek, a tricky little creek not far from downtown Anchorage. We mostly stayed dry but I was often the victim of sweepers, submerged stumps, or sharp turns. I learned pretty quickly how to deal with being upside down in cold water—a skill that turned out to be a lifesaver.

It would be years before I would find out how much being in cold water will accelerate a drop in blood sugar. When you're in cold water in Alaska, you're usually working hard to get out of it. That intense exercise plus your body's burning of all available glucose to try to rewarm itself results in very quick blood sugar drops.

By the summer of 1973 I was ready for bigger, more adventurous trips. At that time the biggest canoe race around was the Kenai River Canoe Race from the Moose River down to the Soldotna Bridge about three hours downriver. With great optimism, I signed up to race with my softball buddy and canoeing partner, Steve Huff, a strong, lean, fiery, athletic guy.

Since the race was on a Sunday, I talked my friend, Bob Campbell and his girlfriend, Bev Koski, into joining Mary and me. We planned to head down to the Kenai Peninsula a day early. The plan was to camp out at the Granite Creek campground on Friday night, canoe down the East Fork River on Saturday, then meet Steve at the junction of the Moose and Kenai Rivers on Sunday for the big race.

Bob trusted me but was inexperienced in canoeing, a bad combination. But he agreed to go. Mary, who had been upside down with me a number of times in Campbell Creek, was smart enough to ask what I knew about the East Fork. I candidly told her "Nothing," except where it was. She offered as how it might be a good thing to ask someone about it before we went.

That spring I had met a guy who was president of the Knik Canoe Club, a club that has since dissolved either for alliterative infractions or the doling out of bad advice. So I called him for advice. "The East Fork?" he pondered. "Well, I don't know too much about it. I don't think many people have done it since those two guys died three years ago. But," he declared with the authority of someone who's supposed to have an answer, "you won't have any problem as long as you take out at the bridge." I dutifully reported back to Mary that he had said, "You won't have any problem," but I neglected to tell her about taking out at the bridge.

So Friday afternoon the four of us headed down to the Kenai Peninsula in my VW van with my canoe on top. We found a good campsite by the creek and enjoyed the night around the campfire with no fear of the days ahead.

The next day broke sunny and clear, a little crisp in the early morning but clearly warming. The sunny morning was surely a harbinger of good things to happen on that beautiful Alaskan summer day. We cleaned the campsite and got the canoe ready to launch. The day had warmed to the mid 60s by midmorning so Bob and I removed our jackets and put them on the floor of the canoe.

That morning I had taken a shot of long-lasting insulin and eaten a campfire breakfast of sausage and eggs and bread. After breakfast, I ate one Hershey bar and took one more with me as a precaution against low blood sugar. That was probably overkill but without the ability to test my blood sugar, I had no idea what my starting level was and no idea what was ahead. The only safe thing to do was to make sure my blood sugar was high.

The plan was that Bob and I would head downstream and the girls would meet us in the VW van at the bridge—the one the president of the canoe club had identified as the critical takeout point. As we were getting ready to launch, Mary, in a move that would ultimately prove crucial, tossed two life jackets to us and said, "You better put these on." Bob, who's about 6 feet tall and weighed about 220 pounds, struggled to get the "too small" life jacket cinched. After working at it for a few minutes, he had just about decided to leave it unbuckled but Bev, showing her feisty side, yelled at him enough that he gave it one last effort and the jacket clicked tightly into place.

With Bob in the bow of the canoe and me steering from the stern, we launched the canoe and headed down the creek for what we expected to be a pleasant experience. The river was quite a bit bigger and faster than Campbell Creek but actually easier as there was more room to maneuver. We were enjoying a beautiful day on this fast-moving, small river when we realized we were approaching the bridge much more quickly than we had anticipated.

Mary and Bev were waiting at the bridge as the canoe approached. But not wanting our experience to end so quickly, we made a last-second decision to go on—*past the bridge.* I yelled to the girls, "We'll meet you downriver at Devil's Canyon." As we passed under the bridge, Bob yelled back to them, "This river's a piece of cake."

The next half hour was pretty peaceful. Then I heard what sounded like a Boeing 707 taking off from Anchorage International Airport. But we were over a hundred miles from there. I looked up at the sky and saw nothing that would indicate thunder. Suddenly, as we rounded a bend, Bob yelled out to me, "Which way?" I saw the reason for his alarm. The river narrowed quickly to a roaring chute of whitewater. Even worse, it funneled straight into a logjam. The right-hand side of the creek bypassed the logjam and bore hard right into a 40-foot-high wall of rock, which caused another 10-foot drop to the left before the creek settled down again.

I yelled out, "Hard right!" and dug my stern paddle in hard on the right side of the canoe. Bob pulled hard on the left side of the canoe with his bow paddle. We started to force the bow to the right. But it was too late. We got the canoe angled in the right direction but the force of the water toward the logjam controlled the moment. The bow hit the first low-lying log in the jam, then skidded up and over the next few logs. The stern dropped and dove toward the bottom with me going under the logjam and Bob flipping backward over my head into the fast-moving, icy-cold current.

I was caught under the logjam—belly-up in the tumult of water, froth, and darkness. I started grabbing for anything that seemed solid. My right hand found a solid log. I clasped the fingers of my left hand into my right hand and held on with both hands, my face pointing upwards. Sucking in a combination of air and froth, I tried to muscle my way upwards and against the current. This was life or death. I struggled, coughing and sucking in froth to reach air and daylight. I didn't think about diabetes. I didn't think about blood sugar. I only thought about breathing.

Grabbing one log at a time, I tried to pull my head above water. My arm muscles didn't hurt. I couldn't feel them. I tried kicking my feet. That did nothing. I knew it had to be all arms if I was going to live. Finally I saw some light. I was gaining on the current. Then I saw blue sky. I pulled myself up and rolled onto the top of the pile of logs and lay there hugging the logs for 10 or 15 seconds.

As I collected myself, I stood up and looked around. No canoe, no paddles, no jackets— and no Bob. I took a few tentative steps on the jumbled logs looking for any sign of Bob. Just then, I saw his head rise from the fast-moving water and then resubmerge. He was caught on an underwater log, facing downstream. The hard-rushing current was forcing his upper body down and keeping his head underwater.

I tried to move quickly on my sluggish, cold legs toward where I had seen Bob. He was trapped under the rushing current about 2 feet away from the logjam. After spending a long couple of minutes in the frigid water under the logjam, my body was not responding. I stumbled a couple of times trying to get over the logs to where Bob was. I lay down on my stomach but still couldn't reach him. The current rushed over him like the rapids over a submerged rock.

Then, once again, Bob forced his head up, resisting the frigid, rushing current. He was yelling loudly over the noise of the rushing water. The only thing I could hear clearly was, "My leg is broken." Bob was clearly worn out from fighting the freezing current. I realized he was about to go under again so I screamed to him, "The next time you come up, force yourself closer to the logjam. It's my only chance to reach you." Before he could respond, he went back under.

I felt helpless as I watched Bob's upper body forced down by the rushing water—just out of my reach. The additional seconds he stayed underwater could only be stealing his strength and making it more difficult for him to force his way closer to my outstretched right arm. Even if he could get close enough, could I move him against the force of the current? Could I get a 220-pound guy with a broken leg up onto the random and uneven logs?

As this was going through my mind, I saw Bob starting to move again. As he raised himself, I watched the water roiling over his shoulders and tunneling down both sides of his head. His head was out of the water. He was trying to roll his body toward me. It was working. He was close enough for me to touch him. With only seconds to act I reached as far as I could. I closed my right hand over the only thing possible to grab, the left shoulder strap of his life preserver. The strap provided a solid handle for my grip. With my pulling and Bob forcing himself away from the underwater death grip of the log, he broke free. But he was immediately at the mercy of the raging current. As his body started to twist, it brought the right shoulder strap of his life jacket within reach of my left hand. I grabbed at it and caught it.

Now I had Bob with both hands but I was lying flat on the logjam. I had no leverage. I was sliding toward the water. I couldn't stop myself. But with my grip acting as a fulcrum the current swung Bob around so that his right side hit the logjam. Since I was holding the life jacket straps, he had both hands free to grab the nearest logs. Now I could let go with one hand and hold onto a solid log. With no feeling in his legs and no help from them, it took the full strength of both our arms to get him up out of the water, onto the logjam and into the blessedly warm sun.

We both lay on the logs recovering before anyone said much. We knew the next issue was Bob's leg. As the sun warmed his leg, he gradually put weight on it. Though he couldn't feel much, he didn't think it was broken. After warming up for about 20 minutes, we began limping downstream.

In the meantime, the girls had been relaxing alongside the creek when both of our jackets and one of our paddles floated by them. They immediately started upstream thinking that we had dumped the canoe and stepped out onto the bank and would be walking downstream. Well, they were certainly right about us dumping the canoe but we didn't exactly just step out onto the bank.

We met the girls and got back to where they had parked the VW van. We presumed the canoe was history. So we headed back to our campsite. We built a roaring fire and told and retold the story to our patient ladies. About 8 p.m. that night another group of canoers came by our site. They had planned a similar route until we told them of our adventure. As it turned out they put in downstream of the logjam and found my canoe—beaten up but not destroyed.

The Sunday race was still on for us. We met Steve at the appointed place and raced in the Kenai Canoe Classic. That race was canceled a few years later when two guys drowned.

A variation of this story first appeared in the book, *Oh No! We're Gonna Die Too* By Bob Bell.

Find your happiness within as you travel on your ways;

Life is what you make it in the story of your days.

—Rick Mystrom (1964)

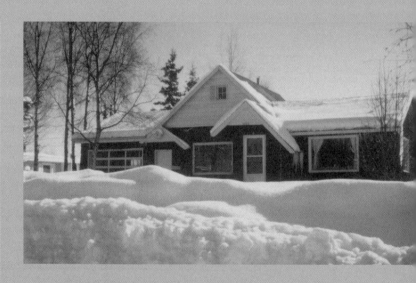

Within a year Mary and I bought our first home in Anchorage.

Chapter 6

Building a Life in Alaska

Sports Opens the Doors

Within my first 10 minutes on the job at KIMO-TV, Rod Hill, one of the other salesmen and a softball player and coach, came up to me and said, "I saw your résumé. It said 'various athletic awards.' You play softball?" "Yup," I volunteered, "I'm a pitcher." It didn't take long to figure that while I was thinking fast pitch, he was talking slow pitch.

It also didn't take long for him to talk me into trying slow pitch with the team he was coaching. I loved the game and connected with the team. The softball community became my first connection with the people of Anchorage. Rod became a close friend and my teammates and their families became Mary's and my first social group in Anchorage. Later they would be supporters and volunteers for my early political campaigns. Rod would go on to promote and grow softball into Anchorage's biggest adult-partic-ipation sport.

In my early years in Anchorage, we were typically playing about 60 softball games a summer including three or four Alaskan tournaments and usually one or two in Oregon or Washington. I also started competing in local football and basketball leagues and in snowshoe racing in the winter and canoe racing in the summer.

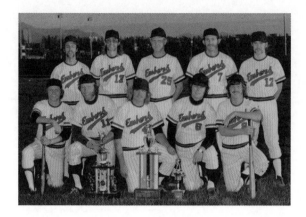

Our softball team was my first group of friends in Anchorage. I'm second from left, kneeling. Rod Hill, second from left standing, Bob Campbell, fourth from left kneeling, and David Haynes, fifth from left kneeling have remained lifelong friends.

Avoiding Low Blood Sugar during Sports or Competitions

In the earlier years before self-testing, I developed a habit that kept me from ever having low blood sugar episodes in those sports competitions. It was, very simply, always eating a candy bar before the game or race. Since I couldn't measure my blood sugar, eating some sugar-filled snack was the only safe thing to do, as I saw it. A chocolate bar was good because it has both sugar and fat. The fat in the candy bar slows the impact of the sugar and helps it last longer. As elementary as the system was, it worked and obviously didn't negatively affect my health much since the only measurable degenerative effect I have from diabetes after nearly 50 years is a slight loss of feeling in my feet.

Although I survived 16 or so years of keeping my blood sugars high to avoid any lows during competition, no one has to do that now. Self-testing gives every insulin-dependent diabetic the opportunity to know exactly where his or her blood sugar is immediately prior to competition and eliminates the necessity of keeping blood sugars unnecessarily high.

Since self-testing, my pattern has been to always try to start a competition or physical activity with my blood sugar between 175 and 200. It protects me from the more urgent and dangerous problem of low blood sugar. It also allows me to focus on the competition and not be distracted by the possibility of a low blood sugar incident.

If my blood sugar is below 175, I'll keep chocolate or Skittles handy. If my blood sugar is above 200 I may give myself a very small bolus (shot) of insulin. But before you decide to give yourself a precompetition shot of insulin you have to determine if your blood sugar is on its way down or on its way up. Insulin on board will lower your blood sugar and food on board will raise it. You must also keep in mind that the competition or the activity will add to the impact of the insulin and will, of course, lower your blood sugar faster than inactivity. In general, you must be very careful about taking a bolus before exercise or competition. If you do give yourself insulin before the activity, my recommendation is that it should be only one half of your normal shot for whatever your blood sugar level is.

In my companion book, *The New Diabetic Lifestyle*, four chapters are devoted to blood sugar control, including a chapter titled, "Sports, Activities, and Blood Sugar Control for Insulin-Dependent Diabetics".

In all my recreational and competitive sports activities, only golf and waterskiing have brought about serious low blood sugar episodes. Golf caused me the most problems until I finally realized how many calories—and therefore how much glucose—a five-hour round of golf can burn even when you're using a golf cart. Waterskiing can be a problem for me because in a water environment I'm not as attuned to the subtle feelings of my body as I am in a land environment. The blood sugar problem is exacerbated for any insulin-dependent diabetic because being in cold water will drop blood sugar very fast as the body uses available energy to try to keep warm.

For the first 10 years I lived in Anchorage, self-testing wasn't available. At that time I was taking one

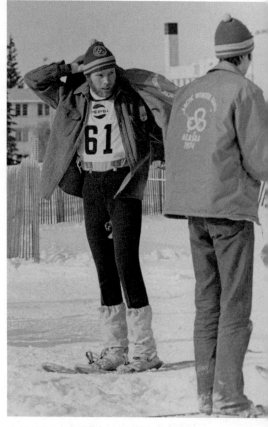

Preparing for the snowshoe race finals in the 1974 Arctic Winter Games.

shot a day of long-lasting protamine zinc insulin. I didn't mix it with any faster-acting insulin so it probably wasn't the best program but it was very predictable. Using avoidance of lows as a measure of success, it was successful. I didn't have an extreme low blood sugar episode in Alaska for about eight years.

A Little Idea That Created a Big Career

My job at KIMO TV started blossoming very quickly. While going out on training with other salesmen, I quickly realized what the biggest barrier to their sales was. It was simply that the owners of the businesses had no idea what they would do with the airtime. If a small company bought one of our packages of 30 commercial breaks of 60 seconds each, they had to figure out how to produce something to put on the air. Most of the businesses the KIMO salesmen called on were small and didn't use an advertising agency. So they just didn't buy TV ads.

After a week of training, I was on my own. The owner sent me to the little towns of Wasilla and Palmer about 40 miles from Anchorage. I guess he thought if I blew my presentations there nobody in Anchorage would know. Besides, nobody had ever sold any TV ads in those little towns so I could get my feet wet with no risk to the station's reputation or revenue.

I called on a few of the larger businesses in the area. One of the businesses was a Ford dealer dealership, Hartley Motors. On the drive out there I came up with this little jingle:

> Drive a little, save a lot.
> Come to Hartley's friendly spot.
> Friendship's high but Fords are not.
> Come to Hartley Motors.

I actually sang it in the shop for the owner, a salesman, and a few mechanics. Not exactly Lady Ga Ga. More like a rough imitation of Tennessee Ernie Ford. But they loved it and signed a year's contract to advertise on KIMO using that jingle. I was onto something that really worked at that time in Anchorage. With success in selling ads using my first jingle, I started coming up with slogans, doing elementary storyboards and writing more jingles for prospective customers in Anchorage. Pretty soon I was selling more than $10,000 a month in ads which gave me over $1,500 a month in commissions, far surpassing my $1,000-a-month expectation.

I continued conceiving and writing ads for my potential customers and soon was selling more air time than any of the other salesmen. I was actually acting a little like an advertising agency but didn't know that at the time.

Within six months I was doing well enough for Mary and me to buy a small, two-bedroom home in the Spenard area of Anchorage. It was our first venture into real estate. The house cost $34,600. Our payment was just over $300 a month and my mom thought we were nuts to pay that much for a house. She and dad had bought our three-bedroom family home in Garden Grove, California 15 years earlier for $9,999 at 3 percent interest with a loan payment of $67 a month.

Mary and I loved our little house. The bedrooms were only about 8 by 10 feet with no room for a dresser, so we kept our clothes in boxes in the hall. Our bed was a foam pad from my Volkswagen van. After we had been in the house about three months, we invited some friends over for our first Thanksgiving in Alaska. We used a door on cinder blocks for a table and sat on the floor. Mary cooked a wonderful dinner and to this day it's one of our fondest Thanksgiving memories.

While I continued to have success selling ads for KIMO, I was frustrated by organizational problems at the station. Ads didn't get on the air. Orders sat on desks. Commercials ran in the wrong slots. About that time, Paul Brown, the advertising manager for the *Anchorage Daily News*, the small, struggling, number-two newspaper in Anchorage, offered me a job as the classified advertising manager for the paper. It was a small increase in pay but offered some incentives if I could grow the classified section. I took the job.

The classified section was eight pages at the time and increasing it to 16 pages would give the *Daily News* a desperately needed boost in revenue and me a nice increase in salary. But there were challenges. When I showed up my first day about eight in the morning I found no one in the office. I went back to the press room and found half a dozen employees with coffee cups in their hands and concern on their faces watching some guy named

Larry trying to get the old, second-hand press cranked up. With a wrench in his right hand, a wrinkled piece of paper in his left hand and grease covering his face so completely that only his two eyes were visible, it was clear to me the fate of that day's paper rested more with him than with the publisher or the editor. The press had broken down and the paper had not been printed—a disaster for a newspaper. He finally got the press fixed and that morning's paper came out by two that afternoon.

During my first week on the job as classified manager, I decided to find out how our classified ads were working for our customers. I started randomly calling the phone numbers in the ads. I very quickly came to three very surprising conclusions: First, most people didn't even know their ads were still in the paper; second, they weren't getting any calls on their classified ads; and third, only about 25 percent of the customers were getting billed for the ads. Wow—eight pages and only the equivalent of two were being paid for.

It took my small staff of three about a week to get all the nonpaying, noncurrent, ineffective ads out of the paper. By the time we had finished, I had succeeded in bringing the classified pages of the *Anchorage Daily News* from eight pages to two pages. Not the direction I had expected. I had some work to do.

We started four or five concurrent promotions. My favorite was the double-time guarantee. If your ad didn't work the way you expected, tell us and we'll run it again for double the length of time you originally ordered. I started making personal calls to realtors and car dealers. We started a number of contests and we brought life and attention to the *Daily News* classifieds.

Within six months our paid classifieds went from two pages up to six pages with everybody actually paying. It was a nice boost for the paper but not enough. The paper was losing money and was unsustainable. The publisher, Kay Fanning, and the general manager, Dave Stein, recognized that their only option for survival was to enter into a joint publishing agreement with their rival, the *Anchorage Times*. The result would be that the whole advertising department would be dissolved and the *Times* would handle the advertising for both papers.

I was not aware of the impending joint publishing agreement but co-incidentally, on a ski slope, I happened to run into the general manager and part owner of my first employer, KIMO-TV. We rode the chairlift together for a few runs where he told me that the sales manager of KIMO had quit. By the end of our third run, he offered me a job as sales manager at KIMO. Both Kay Fanning and Dave Stein encouraged me to take the job without revealing to me that the *Daily News* advertising department would soon be dissolved. I ended up back at KIMO for about two years. I don't recall any spectacular successes in that job but it was during that time I started getting more involved and becoming fairly well known in Anchorage.

Starting Big Brothers of Anchorage

I had been a Big Brother in the Big Brothers program of Los Angeles and had such a good experience I thought I'd like to be a Big Brother in Anchorage. I couldn't find any contact information in the phone book so I called the national Big Brothers headquarters in Philadelphia. They ex-plained that Alaska was the only state in America without a program and would I like to start one. After some discussion with Mary, I agreed to try. I persuaded a few of my friends, including Rick Barrier, Doug Dicken, Jerry Gillian, Bob Todd, Bob Campbell, and Sterling Taylor to join Mary and me in trying to get a Big Brothers program started in Anchorage.

After about a year, we succeeded in getting it started and began making matches. Now, nearly 40 years later it's the statewide "Big Brothers, Big Sisters of Alaska" program with matches in 30 communities around Alaska. The program to date has matched nearly three thousand young Alaskan boys and girls with mentors who have made a positive difference in their lives and according to Tabor Rehbaum, the current program leader, "Rick Mystrom changed what it means to grow up in Alaska."

Getting a Little Complacent about Diabetes

It was 1974 and we had lived in Alaska a little less than two years. Convenient self-testing of blood sugar was still about six years away. I had had no severe lows so it was very easy to get complacent about diabetes. As noted earlier, I'm sure the reason for not having any severe low blood sugar reactions was simply because my blood sugars were probably pretty consistently high. Those patterns of consistently high blood sugars are now firmly established as the primary cause of diabetic complications. But I was young, active, and by almost every physical measure, I was very healthy. I had never taken a sick day in 10 years at any of my jobs. In fact it would be 24 more years before I ever took my first official sick day. That was my last year as mayor when I broke my big toe. I missed two days before I was fitted with a walking cast and returned to work.

By then I had had diabetes for 10 years. I had no symptoms or degenerative problems such as neuropathy or kidney failure. I had no vision problems and no evidence of aneurisms or neovascular growth in the capillaries of my eyes. Nor did I have any evident circulation problems. So even though I did have a few moderate low blood sugar reactions, I was getting pretty complacent in my attitude toward diabetes.

Had it not been for the coming development of blood sugar self-testing and the almost concurrent development of the insulin pump, my life and my health might have been dramatically different. Mary observed once that she thought that the testing devices were more important than the insulin pumps. After 30 years with both, I think she's right. Insulin-dependent diabetics can live a healthy life without an insulin pump by giving themselves frequent shots but they cannot live a healthy life without frequent use of blood sugar testers. It's best to use both but if you choose to only use one, use the self-tester.

Our Second Son, Richard, Is Born

About that time our second son, Richard Tennyson, was born. I had just turned 30 and in those days I still felt that it was more likely than not that I would have some debilitating health problems before I was 40. But that was still 10 years away. Diabetes was still the most common cause of blindness, amputations, kidney failure, and one of the major causes of early death. I remember watching Richard sleep in a little wooden cradle I had made and thinking when he was 10 years old I might not be able to play catch with him, take him fishing, or even watch him play sports. I might not see him graduate from high school, go to college, and probably would not be alive to see him get married unless I recommitted myself to the best diabetic care possible with the technology available at that time.

We now had two sons. For the first time I began believing that with a lot of commitment I could beat the odds. I could be healthy for the biggest part of their lives. I began thinking about all the joy Mary and I would share as they explored and learned about the world beyond our home. It was a time of renewed commitment. I could now clearly see the wonderful times ahead if only I would embrace the healthiest lifestyle possible. I would have to re-commit myself to fully understand diabetes and to learn everything I could about how every different food or combination of foods impacted my blood sugar and therefore my health. Once self-testing became available I spent so much time testing and analyzing my blood sugars that Mary once said to me, "If they ever find a cure for diabetes, you'll have to find a new hobby."

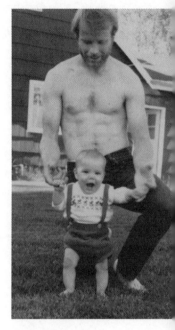

Our second son, Richard, brought squeals of joy to our life daily, and to me a recommitment to healthy living.

Richard's birth gave me that commitment and it was reaffirmed a year later when Nick, our older son, and I were walking in the woods near our house. He was four at the time. We were holding hands as we walked. He was quieter than usual. Suddenly he stopped, looked up at me, and with a quizzical look asked, "Dad, who do you think is stronger? Muhammad Ali, the Six Million Dollar Man, God, or you?"

Well, even fourth place in that group isn't too bad. But it was a moment that made me realize how young sons see their fathers. It made me realize how important it was that I always be there for Nicky and Richard. It was a simple little question from a little boy who thought his dad might be the strongest man in the world. I've never forgotten that question and I've never forgotten how it made me realize how indispensable I was to their young lives.

My complacency about diabetes was gone. I was committed to living a long, healthy life.

Success should be fun.

—Mystrom advertising philosophy

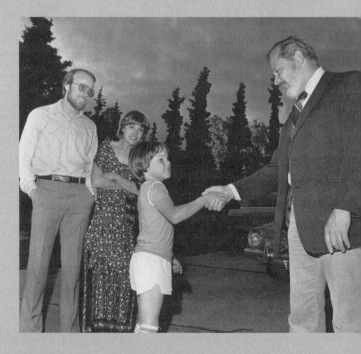

Governor Hammond, following a fund-raising
event at our home for his 1978 re-election
campaign, greets our son, Nick, who just
got home from a soccer game.

Chapter 7

A Growing Business, a Caring Doctor, and Alaskan Politics

My Early Years in the Advertising Agency Business

In late 1974, Larry Beck, a well-known Alaskan entertainer, television personality, poet, and advertising agency owner approached me with a job offer. He had so many different creative endeavors competing for his time that his ad agency, Larry Beck and Associates, was struggling. He offered me the position of vice president of his ad agency. Though it sounded good, I was really the number three person in a five-person company. He was the chairman, his wife, Carol, was the president, and I would be the VP. We also had an art director and a secretary.

It felt like a good fit to me. I liked the creative part as well as the selling, and besides, I'd get a bump in salary and a company car. The construction of the Trans-Alaska Oil Pipeline would soon be underway. People were moving into Alaska and I saw great growth opportunities. I took the job and followed my KIMO pattern of preparing ad concepts, copy, and songs before I even talked to prospective customers. That was an unusual, nontraditional approach for an ad agency, but it was a good strategy for someone who didn't have a history in the business to use as a selling tool. It worked. I began bringing in new clients right away.

I had found a career that I loved. I'd run up the stairs two at a time every morning because it was so much fun to face the day's challenges. Though I loved going to work, I also enjoyed the weekends and all the activities they would bring. I came to the conclusion that if you love Monday mornings as much as you love Friday afternoons you are one of the lucky people who have found balance in life. I had found that balance.

After a few months of watching how unfocused Larry's company was and how busy he was with all his projects, I suggested to him that we divide the company into two different divisions: the advertising division and the "everything else" division. Everything else would include poetry, books, TV programs, and live on-stage entertainment for Alaska tourists. It was what Larry did best. He would head that division and I would head the advertising division. He agreed. So we divided the company just that way.

The advertising division started growing fast and hiring more employees. I told new employees I would offer them "the opportunity to succeed and the freedom to fail." It was up to them to ensure that they didn't fail. We weren't a big company and we couldn't carry people who weren't contributing to our goals. I also told them that I knew how important families and free time were and I didn't expect or even want them to work 50 or 60 hours a week unless we had some extraordinarily important deadline.

Our philosophy was, "Success should be fun"—and it was. We found lots of good reasons for celebrations and parties. In March 1975 we swept all the major advertising awards at the Press Club banquet. We got involved, as a company, in a lot of community service organizations and we competed against other media companies in softball and basketball. Everyone was having fun.

Later that year Larry Beck suggested we split the operation into two separate companies. One company would be Mystrom-Beck Advertising and we would be 50–50 partners in that company. I would be president. The other company would continue to be called Larry Beck and Associates and Larry would continue to do all his projects through that company. He would move Larry Beck and Associates out of our existing office to free up room for Mystrom-Beck's anticipated growth.

I clearly remember Larry and me meeting with a lawyer—his name was Steve DeLisio—to discuss the legal details of the creation of this new company. Steve turned to Larry and said, "As I understand it, Larry, you own this agency and now Rick will own half. How much is he paying you for it?"

Larry, looking a little perplexed, answered, "Well, we hadn't really looked at it that way." Then he turned to me and said, "How about $500?" It didn't take me long to say, "Okay." And it was agreed. I had bought half of the company for $500.

The next year brought growth and creative success. We had some really good employees in those early years—Dennis Smith, Tom Hoffman, Daryl Hoflich, Nita Hopper, David Haynes, and Elaine Huber in our creative department; Marsha Wilson in media; Sue Engman, Linda Boocheever, Mary Cartwright, and Pete Aadland as account executives. Those employees along with our head bookkeeper, Wanda Galyan, all contributed greatly to our early success.

Toward the end of 1975, Mystrom-Beck Advertising had begun to accumulate hefty (by my modest standards) retained earnings. I suggested to Larry that we buy a building. Our existing office above a drugstore, across from a bowling alley, and next to a massage parlor wasn't exactly the high-rent district.

Larry considered it overnight. The next day he said, "Instead of buying a building, why don't you buy me out?" After some negotiations, I did buy him out for $120,000. A bit of a jump from the $500 I had paid for the first half of the company a year earlier, though that first half may have been a tad underpriced. We were now Mystrom Advertising and about to experience some very healthy growth as the price of oil—the driver of Alaska's economy—would soon triple.

Our Third Child

The year 1976 brought another wonderful event, the birth of our third child and our only daughter. Mary wanted to name her Norma or Sara. I thought both of those were too earthy. I figured if I went to the other end of the spectrum, we'd compromise in the middle. So I suggested—with tongue firmly in cheek—Trixie or Flossie. It worked. We settled on Jennifer.

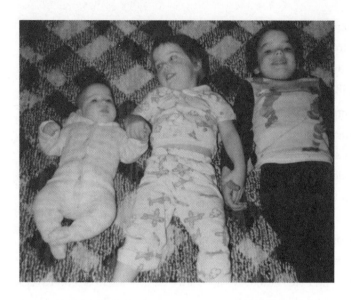

Nick and Rich loved having a little sister from the start. That love among the three has lasted for their whole lives. They are now best friends as adults.

Jenni brought a sense of softness to our rough-and-tumble two-boy family, but more than that, she brought a personality that continually made us laugh with her, at her, at ourselves, and all together. She was a joyous gift to our family. The boys had a little sister to take care of, Mary had the daughter of her dreams, and I had even more reason to stay healthy.

The Importance of a Smart, Involved, and Caring Doctor

Having a good doctor you can learn from, talk to, and confide in is indispensable for a diabetic. I can't conjure up how I first connected with Dr. Jeanne Bonar but I've been her patient, her student, and her admirer for about 35 years now. Dr. Bonar first got me on the pump in 1981, about 32 years ago.

My recollection was that I was the first person to go on the pump in Alaska. When she first suggested it I was hesitant but she persuaded me to try it with a beautifully clear piece of simple logic. "Try it for a month or two," she said, "and if you don't like it you can go back to giving yourself shots." It was simple, logical, and persuasive. I tried it and I've been on a pump ever since.

I remember that same straightforward clarity when she was checking on me in the hospital after one of my extreme low blood sugar episodes.

After one of the four or five times I've been taken to the hospital in Anchorage unconscious with extreme low blood sugar, Dr. Bonar and I discussed exactly what I had done to trigger the problem. In the particular case I'm recollecting, it was after I had been using *both* the pump and a glucose tester. I told her that I had been confident that my blood sugar was high so I gave myself a pretty big infusion without measuring. She reminded me that two of my three previous emergency problems had been caused by that same action: taking a shot without first measuring. She very simply and emphatically said, "Don't do that anymore." She also had a lot more detailed advice that day but I'll never forget that simple command.

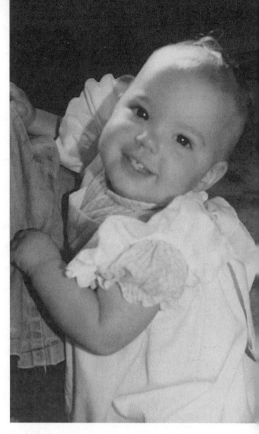

Jenni brought us a sense of softness and joy as she completed our family.

Now when I'm tempted by convenience or haste to just give myself an infusion of insulin without testing, I recall that straightforward bit of advice and test first. That single action has dramatically reduced my low blood sugar reactions. In fact, as I write this, I haven't had an extreme low blood sugar reaction requiring a trip to the emergency room in nearly 20 years.

Nowadays, Dr. Bonar and I talk more like equals. She brings to the discussion the medical and chemical background that I don't have as well as a lot about the new technology and research. I bring to the discussion patient perspective information which comes only from living the experience. But no matter how good your doctor is, you're the one who has control of your own health.

Often in speeches I compare dealing with diabetes to learning to fly a plane. Your instructor may teach you how to fly. But after you've developed the basic knowledge, learned to apply that knowledge, and had a sufficient amount of time flying with your instructor, you're going to fly solo. Your instructor is not going to be with you to tell you how to react in the multitude of situations you'll face, so you need to continually focus on learning and practice. The more you fly the more confident you will become in taking the actions and making the adjustments necessary for your own safety.

Diabetes is similar. You need your doctor to teach you the fundamentals of diabetes, to help you learn the basics of maintaining healthy blood sugar levels, and to get you on a path to better health. But he or she isn't going to walk down that path with you every day. You've got to walk it on your own. The support of parents, siblings, children, or friends will help and regular visits with your doctor or other health care professionals will also help, but like a pilot, you're flying this plane called diabetes. You're the pilot.

Throughout our patient/doctor relationship, Dr. Bonar and I have spent countless hours talking about diabetes generally and my condition specifically. Her leadership in helping me understand and deal with diabetes is a major reason I have had such a healthy life with diabetes. A good relationship with a caring, informed doctor is a great asset in living a healthy life with diabetes.

The Possibility of Pilot Error—Even with a Pump and Self-Testing
Every low blood sugar reaction I have ever had is a result of my errors (I call it pilot error). I've never had a low blood sugar reaction that has been caused by a faulty insulin pump or by faulty glucose measurement that caused me to inject or infuse too much insulin. This book and my companion book, *The New Diabetic Lifestyle*, will help you learn how to be a better pilot. You're the one who has to make the decisions and take the action. Although you need to be vigilant, you don't have to let diabetes dominate your life—but you can't forget it either.

My friend Asa has been with me twice when I was brought to an emergency room with extreme low blood sugar. He once asked me, "Why, if the stakes are so high, aren't you more careful about your decisions?" Good question. This was my answer. I'm giving myself about eight infusions a day with my pump. I often give myself an adjusting infusion of insulin as I wake up in the morning, an infusion for breakfast, often an adjustment midmorning, an infusion for lunch, a midafternoon adjustment, an infusion for dinner, maybe an adjustment before bed, and periodically an adjustment sometime during the night. That's eight infusion decisions a day. Sometimes I do a couple more—sometimes a couple fewer. All together that's about 3,000 decisions a year. Even if you're 99 percent correct in your decisions and 1 percent wrong, that's about 30 errors. Some errors may be too little insulin and some may be too much insulin. But somewhere in those errors are a few dangerous overdoses of insulin which will cause immediate and potentially severe low blood sugar reactions.

You are going to make mistakes. You're human. It's important that your loved ones and supporters are not too hard on you and that you're not too hard on yourself for those mistakes. It's also important that you know how to correct the moderate mistakes so they don't become serious or extreme, and that you always have some emergency glucose or sweets handy for the big mistakes. These issues are covered in detail in my companion book, *The New Diabetic Lifestyle*.

The Importance of Taking Control of Your Life as a Diabetic

Being a well-known diabetic in Alaska has resulted in my being approached by many people with questions or observations about their experience with diabetes. One of the most common observations from diabetics who have *not* taken control of their disease, is that when they're having blood sugar control problems they won't make adjustments until the next time they see their doctor to ask for permission to raise or lower their insulin dosage or change their eating patterns.

Years ago an insulin-dependent Type 1 diabetic who'd had diabetes for about eight years, told me he was getting blood sugar readings in the neighborhood of 300 mg/dl much of the time. He was feeling very lethargic and a little sick to his stomach but was hesitant to change anything. He said his doctor was in Africa and wouldn't get back for a month.

I told him not to let his blood sugars hang around that level for a month. I suggested that he start increasing his insulin dosage a couple of units at a time and keep measuring at the same intervals. "You'll gradually see your readings get lower," I reassured him. I also told him another—and better—option was to eat fewer starchy carbs. He'd see lower readings by doing that too. Now this was a smart guy. He had a responsible management-level job. But unfortunately, I didn't persuade him. No way was he going to change anything until he talked to his doctor. Regrettably, he died a few years ago of diabetes-related complications.

On a more positive note, there was Tony Mattingly, a friend of my sons, who had moved from Alaska to Michigan. He had lost his job in 2009 (along with about 10 million other Americans), so he left his family in Michigan and moved back to Alaska to try to find work. I hadn't seen him in maybe 20 years but he called me one day and told me his 13-year-old son, who was living in Michigan with his mother, had just been diagnosed as a Type 1 diabetic. I invited him to meet me for a cup of coffee so I could give him some background on living with diabetes. He was concerned, interested, and thoughtful. I then invited him to our house the next Saturday to set up a conference call to his wife in Michigan. We talked for about an hour and she too was very interested and involved.

About a month later, he called back and said his son had started football practice in a youth football league and he was having trouble keeping his blood sugar up. Following their doctor's orders, he was taking a shot before an early dinner, then going to practice. According to Tony, his blood sugar was continually getting low during practice. He would regularly have to sit down on the sidelines and try to bring his blood sugar up by drinking colas or eating candy bars until according to Tony, "he couldn't eat any more." I asked Tony how many units his son was taking before meals and he said, "The doctor has him on sixteen units of regular insulin before dinner."

Well, 16 units is a lot of insulin for a young, active kid. I'm certain, however, that the doctor wasn't considering a football practice after dinner. Now 16 units before dinner may have been okay for his usual routine—if there is a usual routine for a teenager—but it was far too much insulin on board preceding a two-hour football practice.

I suggested to Tony that the next time he saw his son's doctor he tell him what had been happening but in the meantime cut his son's shot before practice down to about eight units and see how that worked. I told him if

I had a son his age with insulin-dependent diabetes, I would much rather have him start practice at 200 mg/dl than at 100. When a young boy like that is out playing football it's much more important to focus on avoiding low blood sugar rather than worrying about high blood sugar. Let him play football without worrying about a low reaction. Let him go out there and be a boy. Let him have fun without worrying about diabetes. Now I don't know if Tony and his wife followed my advice or not but I'm guessing they did because of their interest and willingness to learn. I'll also bet that their son is enjoying football more and is more likely to continue with more athletic activities and be healthier by doing so.

Certainly, some people reading this book are saying, "He's not a doctor, how can he advise someone to change insulin dosage?" Well, every day all over America, diabetics are talking with one another, giving advice, asking for advice, telling about experiences, and just generally learning from each other. The more they communicate the better they become at knowing what to expect, what to try, and what to reject. Those discussions are going on all over America—and probably the world—and it's making us all healthier.

You can't do it without a good doctor to get you started and help you along. But he or she can't anticipate the universe of situations you'll face. You've got to make the decisions that will enable you to live a long, healthy life with diabetes.

Governor Hammond and My Introduction to Alaska Politics
By late 1977 Mystrom Advertising had grown to about 20 employees. We had a bank, an airline, a hotel, a lumber company, a grocery chain, an oil company, and maybe two dozen other Alaska-based businesses as clients. We swept the statewide advertising awards that year and were enjoying financial success but the most career-changing event that year originated from a letter I sent to Alaska's governor, Jay Hammond.

Governor Hammond was running for reelection and I liked what he had been saying on the radio and on TV, as well as how he was saying it. He was strong, charismatic, and articulate. He was a pilot, a poet, a commercial fisherman, and a former legislator. He was pure Alaskan, more comfortable in a flannel shirt than he was in a sport coat or God forbid, a tie. He was someone I could commit to support.

In November 1977, the year preceding the election, I wrote a concise, two-paragraph letter to him. The first paragraph said simply that I owned an advertising agency and that we would like to do the advertising for his campaign. In the second paragraph, I said if his campaign already had an advertising agency, I would offer my services as volunteer for his campaign.

Within a week, I got a reply from Governor Hammond. It was hand-written on a piece of plain white paper. He thanked me for the letter and said he had asked Bill McConkey, his campaign manager to contact me. Within a matter of days I met with Bill, Larry Holmstrom, a film producer, and Eric Sanders, a bright young attorney. They were key players on the governor's campaign team. Very shortly after those meetings I got a call from Bill saying that Mystrom Advertising would be part of the campaign team. They wanted us to produce all the brochures, flyers, newspaper ads, and signs, and do all the media buying.

Three days later Bill, Larry, and I were on a flight to Juneau for an evening meeting with the governor at the Governor's Mansion. The three of us met with the governor for little more than an hour. He was every bit as charismatic in person as he was on radio or TV. He was relaxed, friendly, and happy to be out of his tie, which he called "the most damnable idea ever foisted upon the western world."

The meeting wasn't so much a strategy session as it was a motivational pep talk. The governor talked more about Bob Atwood, the publisher of the *Anchorage Times*, the largest and most influential newspaper in the state, than he did about his opponent in the Republican primary, Wally Hickel. The *Times* was an unwavering supporter of Wally Hickel and his "full speed ahead" development philosophy.

Atwood's support plus the fact that Wally Hickel had an extraordinary record of business success made him not only a formidable foe but also a 20-point leader out of the box in the primary race. Wally was a former governor, former Secretary of the Interior under President Nixon, one of Alaska's largest developers, as well as owner of the Captain Cook Hotel and a number of shopping centers in Alaska. He was also very popular in Anchorage, Alaska's largest city.

At that meeting I remember Governor Hammond telling the three of us very eloquently but very concisely why he thought his reelection was important for Alaska. He talked about a range of issues but I recall specifically his concern that when the construction of the Trans-Alaska Pipeline was complete, Alaska would likely see a loss of jobs and possibly an enduring recession. He didn't have specifics but he was committed to finding a way to avoid the impending job losses. He didn't mention the creation of an Alaska Permanent Fund—a fund created by Governor Hammond and the legislature in 1976 to set aside a percentage of oil revenue from the North Slope oil fields for future generations—in that meeting but it did come up often in later discussions.

Sometime during the meeting, I recall him saying that his philosophy of leadership had always been to surround himself with people who were smarter than he was. As a 33-year-old newcomer to Alaska, I was starting to enjoy the feeling of rising smugness that was fed by that comment—until the governor finished the thought by saying, "Fortunately for me, I have a large field to choose from." That comment was very typical of his endearing, self-deprecating humor.

As the meeting was ending, he looked very directly at each of us and said with absolute confidence and a wry smile, "We're behind by a significant amount right now but with this group of creative alchemists there's no doubt that we'll prevail in this election." I'm not sure if any of the three of us knew exactly what an alchemist* was but it was very clear that he was confident in the team. I walked out of that meeting committed to the campaign and motivated to do everything I could to make it successful.

*I think the definition of an alchemist he was referring to was "a person who is committed to transmuting a substance of modest value to something more valuable."

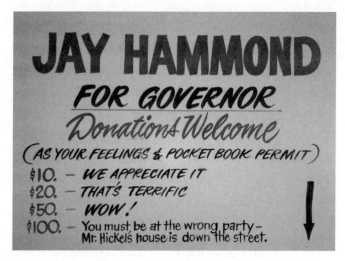

The fund-raising sign at the entry to our home for 1978
reelection fund-raising event for Governor Jay Hammond.
The price of politics has gone up a little in the past 35 years.

The next eight months were an exciting learning experience for all of
us at Mystrom Advertising. We worked long hours, adding our work on
Governor Hammond's campaign to the continually increasing workload
of our growing account list. We were helped immensely by two other key
people: Terry Miller, the popular lieutenant governor and Kent Dawson,
a savvy young Juneau resident with a keen political sense.

As the campaign progressed, we began doing monthly surveys at shopping centers throughout the state. They were pretty unscientific but did
give us a trend line. We increased the frequency of the polls to twice a week
in the last month of the campaign. We had been slowly and consistently
narrowing Wally's lead. With two weeks left, our polls still showed Hammond
slightly behind. It wasn't until the Sunday before the primary election that
our polls showed him holding a slight lead.

With our unsophisticated technique of polling, that lead meant little
else other than that we had closed the gap and the election would be close.
And close it was. When all the votes were counted and the smoke of the
attendant controversies had dissolved, Jay Hammond had beat Wally Hickel

in the primary by 98 votes. He went on to defeat Democrat Chancy Croft in the general election by 16,000 votes.

Wally Hickel accepted the result with dignity and later was elected governor once again. To his credit, he never once mentioned my support of Jay Hammond in any negative way even though he lived just five houses away from Mary and me and often passed our house displaying the only "Jay Hammond for Governor" yard sign in our whole neighborhood.

About 20 years later two other political yard signs in our neighborhood got a lot of attention on national late-night talk shows. In the late '90s Steve Strait ran against Becky Gay for the Alaska House of Representatives, so as you drove through the neighborhood you'd see most of the homes displaying signs in their front yards that said either STRAIT or GAY.

During that time, Mary and I hosted a visiting delegation from Japan. As they drove into our neighborhood, the delegation leader asked their interpreter what the signs were. She told the group she wasn't certain but they appeared to represent the sexual orientation of people in the homes. She further defended her interpretation of the signs by saying that Alaskans were very open about "things like that." It didn't take them long after they arrived in our house to ask us about the signs. It provided us with the icebreaker that made for a very fun reception.

We had been in Alaska for six years. Mary and I had three wonderful, healthy young kids. I had no indications that my diabetes was negatively impacting my health. And we had no indication that any of our kids had diabetes. Richard, though, who was four then, had watched me sometimes eat a candy bar before dinner and thought that maybe diabetes would be a good thing for him to have. Having watched me take shots in my thighs, he pointed to his left thigh and said he thought he had diabetes in that leg, then asked Mary if he could have some candy.

I had learned that I could never forget that I had diabetes but I wasn't letting it dominate my life. I had taken charge of my life and let diabetes come along for the ride.

My business was succeeding beyond all my expectations. I was more and more involved in the community and political office for me was just around the corner.

If you love life then do not waste time;

For that is the stuff life is made of.

—Benjamin Franklin

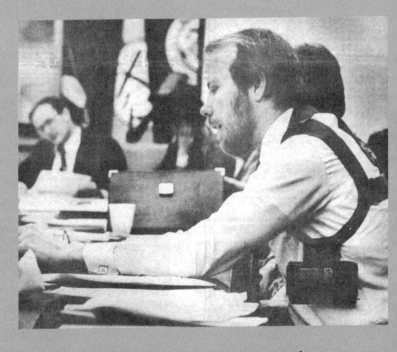

A photo of me at an assembly meeting from a story in the *Anchorage Daily News* about my having the first insulin pump in Alaska. I had a police shoulder holster modified to carry the pump under my arm.

Photo courtesy of Paul Brown, Anchorage Daily News

Chapter 8

Political Office, Extreme Low Blood Sugar, and an Insulin Pump

Winning My First Political Campaign

By early 1979 we had just completed two very successful years with Mystrom Advertising. Mary and I had gotten more and more involved in community activities and I started thinking about running for the Anchorage Municipal Assembly, typically called the city council in other cities.

I had grown to appreciate Anchorage and its people and wanted to get more involved. In retrospectives and memoirs, many politicians often attach a noble purpose to their first run for office. For the life of me I can't conjure up what, if any, noble purpose motivated me to run for the first time. I do, however, know whose influence first planted the political seeds in my mind.

My sister, Rosanne Bader, and her husband, Chuck, got me involved in Chuck's first political campaigns—successful runs for mayor of Pomona, California and later for the California State Assembly. I was also influenced during my college years by the charisma of President Kennedy and the oratory of Martin Luther King. On the Alaska landscape, Governor Jay Hammond, Anchorage Mayor George Sullivan, Assemblyman Dave Walsh, and State Senator Arliss Sturgulewski were also inspirations.

Although Mary and I had lived in Anchorage only seven years, we had a large group of friends who were willing to help in our first political foray.

Because so many people had moved to Anchorage from what Alaskans refer to as "Outside" or the "Lower 48," it had (and still has) a population with few extended families. The absence of extended family connections in Alaska results in the bonds of friendships forming more quickly and lasting longer than in other cities with more extended families. Somehow it didn't seem unusual that I should run for office, even as a relatively short-term citizen of Anchorage.

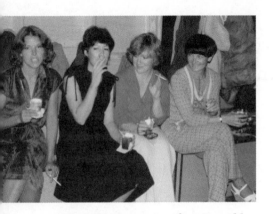

Key volunteers on my first Assembly campaign taking a smoke break in the garage. From left to right, my wife Mary, Jeri Anderson, Kay Steele, and Mary Jones. I hope they're not too mad at me for including this photo in the book.

Each assembly district in Anchorage had about 30,000 people then. Our district, West Anchorage, had two assemblymen, Dave Walsh, a bright young attorney and very much a leader on the assembly, and Bill Besser, who had been in office for 19 years. Bill's term was up in October 1979. I decided to run against him.

Our campaign team consisted of Mary and a few of our close friends: Bill and Jeri Anderson, Lloyd and Kay Steele, Lloyd and Joan Morris, Mike and Tuney Zoske, and Mary and Bart Jones. Also on our campaign team were parents of the youth hockey team I was coaching, and my softball teammates. None of them, by the way, knew anything about political campaigns. But with all the things we did wrong, we must have done some things right because I won in a landslide.

Face First and Unconscious with a Candy Bar in My Hand

It was during the campaign, but not related to it, that I had my first *extreme* low blood sugar reaction in Alaska. Mary and I had just bought a small ski chalet in the town of Girdwood, home to Alyeska, Alaska's largest ski resort, about 45 minutes south of Anchorage. Our family had driven down to Girdwood for our first full-family look at the chalet.

As we were walking around the newly built and completely empty chalet, I began feeling that my blood sugar was getting low. There was absolutely nothing in the chalet and, unbelievably, I was not carrying emergency sweets or glucose with me. With absolutely no sugar or glucose available in the brand-new chalet, I told Mary I was going to drive the mile or so to the mercantile store, locally called "The Merc," and get something to raise my blood sugar. By the time I got to the store, my blood sugar was very low and evidently going down fast. I walked into the store, but my low blood sugar stole my ability to think clearly. My brain needed glucose to function and wasn't getting it.

I walked around the store, confused and not knowing why I was there. I stopped in front of the candy section but still didn't know what I needed. It was the brown wrapper of the Hershey bars that triggered my brain. I started tearing the wrapper off a Hershey bar. That's as far as I got. The next thing I recall was the voice of a paramedic sitting with me in the back of an ambulance. I kept fading in and out of consciousness. We were heading toward Anchorage with Mary and the kids following in her car.

Later that night at the hospital, Mary pieced together the story for me. The clerk had told her that I walked into the store and just ambled around for a couple of minutes as if I didn't know what I was looking for. She then saw me grab a candy bar and try to get the paper off. Before I got the paper off, I fell into the counter then onto the floor and started convulsing. She called 911. The fire station was less than 500 yards away and an ambulance was there within minutes.

As the emergency medical technicians were attending to me at the store, Mary, still in our little chalet with the kids, had started to worry. She loaded the kids in her car and drove to the store. She saw the ambulance and immediately knew what had happened. She talked to the paramedics and then followed the ambulance to the hospital in Anchorage.

That was my third extreme low blood sugar episode requiring emergency care—two in California and now this one in Alaska. It was also the last episode I would have in my pretesting, pre-insulin-pump days.

I have no idea why I was so slow learning to carry some emergency sweets but doing so would have prevented at least half of my extreme low blood sugar reactions requiring hospitalization. No insulin-dependent diabetic, whether Type 1 or Type 2, should ever be away from home without some kind of quick-acting candy or glucose tablets.

I now keep Skittles in my pocket, in my car, in Mary's car, in my golf bag, my fishing box, and my shaving kit. Sometimes I'll carry a packet for months without ever needing it but having them on my person is my security blanket. On a lighter side, I recently gave a talk to an assembly of fifth- and sixth-graders about being mayor and having diabetes. I told them I always have Skittles with me to bring my blood sugar up if needed. I somehow missed the mark in my explanation because most of the very nice thank-you letters written by the students said, "I didn't know Skittles were so good for diabetes."

So I Got Elected—Now What?

I was probably as naïve about politics as most first-time elected officials. I actually thought everyone wanted smaller, more efficient, less costly government. Boy, was I wrong! The Assembly was split with five conservatives, five liberals and one moderate, me. I was in the process of moving more to the conservative side but hadn't completely let go of the liberal influence ingrained in me at the University of Colorado. Not only was I the swing vote on many issues but I was also seated between a quick-witted arch-conservative, Fred Chei, and a smart, likeable liberal, Jane Angvik. They often engaged in acerbic debates that make Nancy Pelosi and Rush Limbaugh seem like valentine sweethearts.

During budget debates in Anchorage, hundreds of people filled the assembly hall to speak out for more government programs or less government spending. Some, amazingly, spoke out for both. It didn't take me long to come to a very revealing and probably pretty obvious way of predicting how people were going to testify. Those people who were primarily tax receivers or associated with tax-receiving groups supported larger city budgets and therefore higher taxes. Those who were primarily taxpayers and not associated with tax-receiving groups supported smaller city budgets and lower taxes.

The same holds true at the national level and probably has ever since federal income tax was first authorized in 1861 to pay for the Civil War. The size and spending of the federal government continues today as one of the clearest philosophical distinctions between Democrats and Republicans.

Politics during the Oil Boom in Alaska

During my first term on the Anchorage Assembly I was earning a reputation, according to the newspaper articles at the time, as "... a moderate conservative and a problem solver." I had been successful at helping keep the cost of government down. Joe Griffith, the assembly budget analyst at that time and now an indispensable statewide leader, said, "No one has been better at getting thoughtful, careful cuts in Anchorage budgets passed than Rick Mystrom."

The construction of the 800-mile Trans-Alaska Oil Pipeline was completed in May 1977 at a cost of $8 billion. It was then, and still is, one of the largest privately funded construction projects in the world. As the construction wound down people and companies were leaving Alaska and the Alaskan economy was slowing. But in 1980, my second year on the Assembly, the price of oil jumped to over $30 a barrel. It had been just over $3 a barrel 10 years before that when the pipeline construction was being planned.

The dramatic increase in the price of oil and the ability to transport oil from the North Slope of Alaska to the deep-water port of Valdez through the Trans-Alaska Pipeline stimulated much more investment by the oil industry in Alaska. It also represented the beginning of a codependent and mutually beneficial relationship between the State of Alaska and the Alaska oil industry.

Because of the royalty and severance taxes paid to the state on every barrel of oil going through the pipeline, the government of Alaska was awash in money in the early '80s. Fortunately, Governor Hammond and the state legislature realized that this was a timely opportunity to develop infrastructure and facilities to improve the economy and quality of life in Alaska.

The governor proposed and the legislature approved a three-year capital improvement program for Alaskan communities, under which the state would grant every community in Alaska $1,000 per citizen every year for three years for capital projects. With Anchorage's 175,000 people in 1980, our city would be getting about $175 million dollars a year for three years—in addition to the usual state funding for annual construction of roads, schools, and public safety buildings.

Under the leadership of Mayor George Sullivan and with the support of the Anchorage Assembly, "Project '80s" was conceived. The mayor proposed and the assembly approved the construction or expansion of four public buildings with these funds. We constructed a sports arena, a convention center, a new library, and a major museum expansion. Later, under the leadership of Anchorage's new mayor, Tony Knowles, a performing arts center and a major road-building program were completed with these funds.

It was during the debate and vote on Project '80s that I lost my biggest assembly battle of my first term. The issue was whether Anchorage should build a multi-use, dome-style sports arena for both recreational and competitive use, or a competition-only sports arena. As a rookie Anchorage assemblyman, I thought a dome-style, multipurpose arena would best serve the people of Anchorage. However, the popular longtime mayor of Anchorage, George Sullivan, wanted a traditional, competition-only sports arena. No contest. Mayor Sullivan won. The George M. Sullivan Sports Arena has served Anchorage well for nearly 30 years now.

This combination of the petroleum industry exploration and production combined with capital projects attracted oil industry service firms, engineering firms, architectural firms, contractors, construction workers, and service workers. It also triggered an influx of banks and savings and loan institutions. The economy and the population of Anchorage boomed. Anchorage benefited hugely because it represented then—and still does now—more than 40 percent of Alaska's population. Only the state of New York has a bigger percentage of its population represented by a single city.

New high-rise office buildings were constructed, large and small apartment complexes sprang up, homes and condos were built and filled as fast as they were finished, and fast food chains discovered Anchorage. Only 65 years old at that time, Anchorage grew from relative youth to gangly puberty during the early '80s.

The boom would last for five years until 1986, when "irrational exuberance" (sound familiar?) in housing construction stimulated by loose lending practices (sound familiar?) combined with the Tax Reform Act of 1986 and a dramatic drop in oil prices to demolish the real estate market and consequently the Alaskan economy.

From the start of the economic collapse in early 1986 to the start of its recovery in 1989, Anchorage would lose 13 percent of its population and see a 25 percent drop in the assessed valuation of all buildings in the city. In 1985 I had seen evidence of overbuilding beginning to surface and spotted a potential recession on the horizon. While I did recognize the overbuilding, I didn't see it compounded by a drop in oil prices. By that time I had purchased eight apartment buildings and a commercial building in downtown Anchorage. The good news was I was prescient enough to sell five of the buildings at the peak of the economy in late 1985. The bad news was I kept four. But we survived financially and never missed a mortgage payment. I kept my credit rating intact and was able to buy more buildings at the bottom of the market.

Living a Busy, Active Life with Diabetes

The economic boom had been a fun, challenging, and busy time on the Anchorage Assembly. In addition to all the assembly work associated with an economic boom, and building my advertising agency, I continued coaching our kids' sports teams. I was coaching Nick's and Rich's teams in hockey, baseball, basketball, and football. Our youngest, Jenni, was just starting basketball and all the parents assumed that I'd coach her teams too. They were right. I began coaching her elementary school basketball team and ended up coaching most of her basketball and softball teams through junior high.

Our kids gave our family so many opportunities to laugh together and at ourselves. I recall one morning as I was getting dressed for work, Nick, who was a freshman at West High School in Anchorage, came into our bedroom and said, "Dad, can I wear one of your shirts to school today?" I answered with fatherly pride, "Sure, Nick. Help yourself." As I went downstairs to join Mary and our other kids at the breakfast table, I mentioned to Mary that Nick was wearing one of my shirts to school that day. She smiled and said, "I know. Today's Nerd Day at West." I think it was my favorite shirt he wore.

As I reflect on all the youth teams I coached—something over 20 teams—and all the teams I competed on since I was diagnosed with diabetes (about 60 teams), I am both pleased and amazed that I never had one severe low blood sugar episode while competing or coaching. I'm sure the reason for that was simple. Before self-testing, I always ate a candy bar before starting. After self-testing, my habit was to always test my blood sugar before competition started.

I adjusted well to being on the municipal assembly, growing Mystrom Advertising, helping Mary raise our three kids, coaching their teams, and still competing in sports myself. Life was good but for me it was about to get much better.

The Technology That Changed My Life

On Monday, November 30, 1981 at eight o'clock in the morning I met Dr. Bonar at Alaska Regional Hospital for an orientation to a newly available device called the insulin pump. As an aside, when I was reviewing my calendars to determine the exact date I got my insulin pump, I had to smile when I looked at Mary's and my schedule for the Saturday before my Monday appointment to get my pump. Here's what it said:

9:45 a.m.	Nicky Basketball
11:30 a.m.	Jenni Hockey
2:00 p.m.	Nutcracker Ballet
6:45 p.m.	Rich Hockey
8:00 p.m.	Nicky Basketball
9:30 p.m.	Festival of Trees

It was a typically busy day for that stage of our lives and obviously a very fun one.

In those days to get a pump you had to check into a hospital. I recall, as the pump's functions were being explained and the pump inserted, quite a few hospital staff members were gathered around to learn about this new device.

I liked my pump from the start. I appreciated its flexibility and the ability to infuse insulin multiple times during the day. The first pumps, however, had a significant void. They had no memory. After a month or so of using the pump I got so accustomed to it, I would give myself an infusion (also referred to as a shot or a bolus) of insulin without even thinking about it. Half an hour later I'd be wondering whether or not I had given myself a shot. But it wasn't long before that flaw was corrected.

My first pump was so big that I went to the "cop shop," a local store for police supplies and asked them to make a custom shoulder holster that held my pump under my arm. I'd always get a lot of murmurs when, at an Assembly meeting, I stood up and took off my suit jacket and revealed the shoulder holster. I'd sit back down and announce to the audience, "Sometimes these meetings get pretty feisty."

But the insulin pump would not have been effective, or even useful, without the concurrent advent of self-testing monitors. The two technologies together represented the biggest advance in diabetic self-care since the invention of insulin by Doctors Banting and Best of the University of Toronto in 1922.

Now for the first time I could get blood sugar readings multiple times every day instead of once every three months or so. And I could react to them by giving small infusions of insulin as needed. The first blood sugar testers involved blotting the blood samples and it took a minute or two for the whole process. Now the process is much simpler and takes about 5–10 seconds.

My First Lesson after Starting Self-Testing

It didn't take me more than a week or so of testing to realize that my blood sugar was high most of the time and probably had been most of my diabetic life. The obvious reason, as I said earlier, was that in the 16 years I'd had diabetes prior to self-testing, my primary goal had been to avoid the immediate dangers of low blood sugar. In avoiding lows, I ended up with pretty consistently high blood sugars. I'm quite certain that was the case with most insulin-dependent diabetics before self-testing was available.

In 1981 many theories about tight control vs. loose control were still being discussed. Two years later a 10-year study called the Diabetes Control and Complications Trial (DCCT) was initiated. The results were so dramatic and revealing that the study was actually concluded after nine years so the information could get out one year earlier. The health advantages of keeping blood sugars as close to normal (75 to 105 mg/dl) as possible were accepted as irrefutable. The tight-control advocates were correct.

The conclusions of the trial as reported by the National Institute of Diabetes, Digestive and Kidney Diseases showed that *intensive control* of blood sugars resulted in a 76 percent reduction in the risk of eye disease; a 60 percent reduction in the risk of nerve disease; a 57 percent reduction in the risk of heart attack, stroke, or death from cardiovascular causes, and a 50 percent reduction in the risk of kidney disease.

Here are the elements of intensive management (or control) as defined by the DCCT:

1. *Testing blood glucose levels four or more times a day*

2. *Injecting insulin at least three times daily or using an insulin pump*

3. *Adjusting insulin doses according to food intake and exercise*

4. *Following a diet and exercise plan*

5. *Making monthly visits to a health care team composed of a physician, a nurse educator, dietitian, and behavioral therapist*

According to the National Diabetes Information Clearing House, the study compared the effect of standard control of blood sugar versus intensive control on the complications of diabetes. Intensive control meant keeping A1C levels as close as possible to the normal value of 6 or less. The A1C blood test is an index which reflects a person's average blood glucose over the last two to three months. Six percent, by the way, is very hard to achieve. My A1C levels since I've been out of public office range from 6.7 to 7.2, which is where Dr. Bonar wants me to be. When I was mayor and had a long and intense schedule, my A1Cs were in the high sevens and low eights, which was not very good.

Of the five elements suggested to represent intensive (or excellent) control, I follow the first four very closely. They suggest testing four times a day. I test six to 10 times a day. They suggest injecting insulin three times a day or using an insulin pump. I use a pump. They suggest following a diet and exercise plan. I do.

The fifth recommendation, monthly visits to a health care *team* consisting of a physician, a nurse educator, dietician, and behavioral therapist is not achievable for the average person. I don't even come close to that. I chalk up a monthly visit with a four-person medical team as an ideal dream but totally unrealistic. If you can afford to visit a four-person medical team every month, God bless you. But most people can't and no insurance company I know of will pay for that, nor will Medicare. Those team visits may be helpful early in your experience with diabetes but consult with your doctor about the most appropriate ongoing frequency of visits and what other medical professionals, if any, can be there.

My First Serious Low Blood Sugar Experience with My Pump

Using an insulin pump does not mean that you will never have low blood sugar episodes. The pump does mean, however, that you will have more control over your insulin infusion, more flexibility in your mealtimes, better blood sugar control, and an opportunity for a healthier life. But your blood sugar control is still dependent on your own decision making.

In Maui, Hawaii in the fall of 1982, about a year after I got my pump, I made a really stupid mistake. Mary and I were playing tennis at our hotel one evening. Because tennis shorts in those days were pretty tight, I had no logical place to put my insulin pump and since that was way before the days of the detachable systems, I decided to detach the pump by removing the syringe from my pump and putting the syringe in my pocket. The syringe cylinder had about three days' supply of insulin in it and was still attached to my body by a tube. I put the syringe cylinder in my tight front pocket of my tennis shorts.

After about an hour we finished our last game and I jumped over the net to give Mary a hug and I instantly felt a big gush of insulin going into my leg. I pulled the syringe out of my pocket and confirmed my fear. It had emptied. I had just infused about three days' worth of insulin into my body. It was at least eight times bigger than the biggest dose of insulin I have ever injected at one time. I now realize that it was very possibly a lethal dose. Without immediate action, I would have gone into a potentially fatal seizure within a half hour.

We ran back to our room and called the hotel staff. They said no clinic was open and no hospital was within 30 miles. They offered to try to contact a doctor. This was Maui in the early '80s and I knew no doctor would be there quickly enough to help. I asked Mary to run to the restaurant and get whatever high-calorie, sugary food she could. I had to offset that huge infusion of insulin. Within 10 minutes she returned with two pies and a large container of orange juice. Once more she came through when she had to.

I knew I had enough sugar to stop the impending deadly drop of my blood sugar, but I also knew it would be the start of a long, uncomfortable night. I would have to eat all that sugary stuff continuously for at least three, maybe four hours to counteract the huge overdose of insulin. I also knew if I fell asleep or threw up I would be in grave danger. I just had to keep shoveling in sugary calories. Mary stayed awake with me the whole time to be sure I didn't fall asleep. I tested my blood every 15 minutes and despite eating what I'm guessing was over 10,000 calories of sweets my blood sugar never got high enough for me to feel that I was safe until somewhere around 2 a.m. Finally I was able to stop. I felt uncomfortably full for about two days. But we did what we had to do and I survived.

My best guess is that I accidentally injected somewhere around 90 units of insulin into my body in that Maui episode. I remember during that critical episode trying to recall the details of news stories of a doctor somewhere in New York who had gone on trial accused of killing his wife with an overdose of insulin. I couldn't recall ever reading how much insulin he had injected into her. Whatever it was, I was quite sure it wasn't as much as I had injected into myself.

All my serious low blood sugar episodes were caused by mistakes I made. All were avoidable and most were understandable. But this one— well, it was just plain dumb.

The important thing in life is not the destination but the journey.

—Anonymous

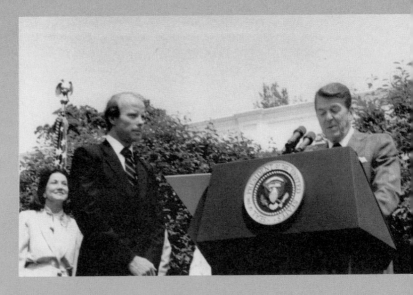

Receiving the award as one of America's top three
Small Businessmen from President Reagan.
Secretary of Transportation Elizabeth Dole
is in the background.

Chapter 9

Lots of Travel with Very Few Blood Sugar Problems

Mystrom Advertising had continued to grow. Both Mary and I were very involved in our community. Our boys were playing on hockey, basketball, soccer, and baseball teams and Jenni was just starting kindergarten. As I was driving her to school one morning she proudly announced that she had decided what she wanted to do when she grew up. I asked her what that was. She said that she was going to be a professor. I told her I thought she'd be a good professor. She smiled at my encouragement and then said, "I'm not really sure. I think I either want to be a professor or a cheerleader." The kids brought Mary and me daily joy in huge helpings. We loved our lives.

I won reelection to the Assembly with a 70 percent majority. I like to think the victory margin was a result of my performance on the assembly but the margin was likely enhanced by my receiving an award from President Reagan as one of the top three Small Business Persons in America.

Into the White House Rose Garden with
My Insulin Pump in a Concealed Shoulder Holster
In 1982 I was selected by the Alaska Small Business Administration as Alaska's Small Business Person of the Year and then as the Top Small Business

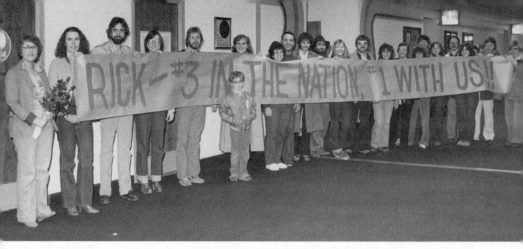

Employees of Mystrom Advertising who really deserved most of the credit for my award greet us on our return from Washington, D.C. Our son Richard is in front.

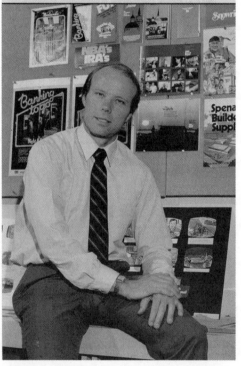

This photo was taken just after I had been selected as the top Small Businessman for Alaska and the Pacific Northwest.

Person in the Pacific Northwest. Soon after that Mary and I got an invitation from President Reagan's social secretary to attend a ceremony in the White House Rose Garden to honor America's Small Business Persons. We took our 10-year-old son Nicky with us to share in the experience.

At that time I was still wearing my large insulin pump in a shoulder holster under my suit jacket. The shoulder holster worked well, since my first pump was about the size of a small handgun. I still marvel that Mary, Nicky, and I went through White House security without so much as a pat-down. Had I had a pat-down I'm sure that would have created quite a stir.

We were escorted into the Rose Garden. Mary was seated in the front row with Nicky on the grass in front of her. The day before, as we toured Washington, I had just given Nicky a little lesson in frugality. He had been using his point-and-shoot camera with abandon and I felt compelled to tell him that every time he pressed the button, it cost about 50 cents including the film and development costs. I told him to be more selective and just take one picture of something, not multiple pictures.

Nicky took that lesson to heart. As I was standing on the Rose Garden podium with President Reagan, Nicky was seated on the grass with a few other children about 10 feet from the President and me. I tried to signal to him to take some pictures. Proud that he remembered our talk from the day before he said loudly enough for the President to hear, "I did, Dad. I already took one." The President laughed and continued his comments. So while I didn't have a big selection of pictures of this event to choose from, the *one* he took turned out great and appears at the start of this chapter.

My Second Term on the Anchorage Assembly

My second term on the assembly was by most media accounts very successful. My most vivid recollections of that term are of one big victory and one big loss.

The big victory was gaining support for a tax cap on city government. I had introduced a spending cap. After a month of discussion, Don Smith, a fellow assemblyman, introduced a tax cap ordinance. He convinced me and four others on the assembly that a tax cap was better. My focus was getting the Anchorage business community behind that ordinance. I began an aggressive round of speeches successfully gaining support for the tax cap. The ordinance passed and has served the Municipality of Anchorage well for over 30 years now.

The big loss I recall was my effort to reduce vacation and sick leave time for city employees. I felt the leave time, which was far greater than in the private sector, was too generous. I recall thinking that since it affected so many employees, the only fair thing to do was to invite all those who were interested to a local school gym, certain that they would agree once they heard my explanation Right? Wrong!

I was accustomed to generally positive reactions to most, if not all of my speeches since I had entered public office. Not this one. The gym was packed and was silent when I walked in. It was silent when I began speaking. It was silent when I concluded. It was silent when I asked for questions and it was silent when I walked out. It was a unique experience talking to a few hundred immobile, nonspeaking people. I smile about it now but I have to admit it was a little disconcerting then. My proposal lost by only eight votes (one in favor, nine against).

International Travel with the Insulin Pump

Japan

Early in my second term our newly elected mayor, Tony Knowles, asked me if I would represent Anchorage at the Conference of Northern Mayors in Sapporo, Japan in February 1982. Attending would be the mayors of Edmonton, Canada; Oslo, Norway; Stockholm, Sweden; Helsinki, Finland; Sapporo, Japan; as well as Harbin and Shenyang, China. The purpose of the conference was to share ideas and solutions to problems that are common to northern cities. I told him I would be happy to do it but wanted to pay my own way since I wasn't the mayor. Mayor Knowles, of course, had no problem with that so it was agreed. I would go. I also made plans to visit the mayor and chairman of the assembly of Chitose, Japan, one of Anchorage's sister cities.

Mary and I took our son Rich with us on the trip. He had just turned eight and was a fun traveling companion for Mary and me. On the way to Sapporo we spent a couple of days in Tokyo and while we were there decided to take the bullet train from Tokyo to Yokohama. Not only did the train travel at over 130 miles per hour but its station stops were done at warp speed compared to American trains. The door openings and closings at the stops were automated and seemed to be about 45 seconds in duration. With hundreds of passengers getting off and an equal or greater number getting on, I began to think Japan was the origin of the expression "going with the flow."

At one of these stops we decided the railcar behind us offered more space and we should change cars at the next stop. At that stop we flowed out with the crowd of purposeful, hurrying Japanese business commuters and walked briskly toward the next car. As Mary and I stepped into the next car, I looked down and realized Rich was not with us. The 10-second "door-closing warning horn" was sounding. I still didn't see him. Mary and I had been pushed away from the door by the surging crowd. Mary screamed for Rich. I tried to push my way back toward the door.

This was before the days of cell phones and I shared Mary's heart-stopping fear of leaving our eight-year-old on a train platform filled with a sea of non-English- speaking people while we barreled at 130 miles per hour toward the next town.

With only seconds left, I knew I wasn't going to make it to the door before it closed. The door started closing. Just then I saw this flash of a kid, waist-high to the flowing Japanese crowd, flying toward the door. He made it to the door and dove headfirst and ankle-high into the car as the door closed. Within seconds the train was back up to 60 miles per hour and within minutes back up to 130, with or without Richard. Fortunately, it was *with* Richard.

This was to be the first of some 40 to 50 international trips I have taken since getting the insulin pump. There is no reason why insulin-dependent diabetics should be apprehensive about international travel. The pump is a wonderful tool for just such occasions.

During the conference in Sapporo I developed a friendship with Wang Hua Chen, chairman of the Standing Committee of the People's Congress of Harbin, Heilongjiang Province, China. Harbin is a *medium*-sized city of about 6 million people in Manchuria in northeast China. One of my first memories of Chairman Wang was his visit to my hotel room in Sapporo to pay respects and ask about Alaska. In a rare oversight the Japanese hosts of the conference did not have a Chinese-English interpreter. However, they did have a Chinese-Japanese interpreter and a Japanese-English interpreter. So our conversation started with him speaking in Chinese to the Chinese-Japanese interpreter. She then spoke in Japanese to the Japanese-English interpreter who then spoke to me in English. My response then went back to Chairman Wang in reverse. It was a curious experience to watch a question working its way toward me and my answer working its way back.

The twice-translated conversation must have worked fine; two years later, Chairman Wang extended an invitation to Mary and me to visit China before it was open to unescorted tourists.

China—before It Was Open to Unescorted Tourists

Chairman Wang said that while the central government of China had invited some American delegations, we would be the first Americans invited to China by the Harbin government and as far as he knew we were the first Americans invited by any provincial or city government other than Beijing.

He would arrange for the vice mayor of Beijing and an official party to greet us upon our arrival at the Beijing Airport. Not only was this protocol but, he explained, it was necessary because we couldn't just walk around Beijing on our own. We would have to have an official of the Communist party and an interpreter with us at all times. After the trip was over I concluded that the role of the party official was to gauge our reactions to China and to give our interpreter guidance in helping persuade us of the prosperity and happiness of China's people.

By that time I had been elected chairman of the assembly and I decided to ask the newly elected vice-chair, Jane Angvik and her husband, former state senator Vic Fischer, to join us. Once again I felt that we should pay for the trip ourselves and not look to the city for any reimbursement. She agreed and the planning went forward. It was a good choice. Jane and Vic were fun traveling companions and represented Alaska well.

Because of our invitation from Chairman Wang, quite a bit of planning took place on the Chinese side including the forming of a fairly large welcoming party of dignitaries scheduled to meet us at the airport in Beijing. This delegation would include our Communist party "guide" and an interpreter who would be with us at all times.

But we didn't make our scheduled flight from Tokyo to Beijing. The SAS flight from Anchorage to Narita Airport in Tokyo was late arriving. SAS personnel whisked us through the airport, to the Air China gate where we were surprised but pleased to see the plane to Beijing hadn't left yet. But then we ran into an immovable barrier in the form of a burly Air China employee who stood at the entrance to the Jetway with his arms folded adamantly against his chest. I think he knew only two English words: "Sorry, full," which he repeated over and over no matter what we said to him. It was pretty clear he didn't understand us but we understood him— we weren't getting on.

After the plane pulled away without us, we finally made some contact with an Air China official who knew a few more English words: "Beijing?— maybe next Monday." This was a Thursday and we were scheduled to return to Anchorage on Tuesday. This wasn't encouraging.

We spent the night in a tiny hotel room near the airport and were committed to finding any route possible the next day to Beijing. After talking to dozens of people trying to find even the most circuitous flights to China, we began thinking that the trip might not happen. Just then we saw a JAL employee running toward us. She said, "Please hurry. Bring your luggage." A chartered JAL flight to Beijing with some empty seats was leaving shortly. We made it. A few hours later we were in Beijing with, of course, no welcoming delegation.

We managed to find a hotel and blunder through the check-in process. The next challenge was to get a taxi to a restaurant. By doing a lot of arm waving, stomach rubbing, and pantomiming, we communicated our wishes to a taxi driver. We knew we got through when he repeated the same signs to us and smiled. We nodded yes and were on our way. When we got to the restaurant the driver parked his cab and came in with us. We thought that was kind of him until he spoke to the owner of the restaurant who took us to a table set for five: Jane, Vic, Mary, me, *and the taxi driver*. We had evidently agreed to buy him dinner too. The restaurant he took us to was called the "Sick Duck" restaurant. As you can imagine we were happy to find out the restaurant got its name because it used to be a hospital.

The next day we wandered around Beijing without a guide or interpreter. It was exactly what we weren't supposed to do. The stares, the murmurs, and the pointing as we moved through Beijing reaffirmed that we were among the first Westerners to walk the streets of Beijing unguided. My height and my sparse blond hair got a lot of attention as people young and old alike pointed and followed us as we walked.

Two things we did caused big crowds to form instantly: making any purchase in a store and taking Polaroid pictures of children. The fascination the Chinese citizens had with a purchase indicated how few people could actually buy something other than food. The magical appearance of a Polaroid picture actually frightened some of the 50 to 70 people who gathered instantly around us pushing and leaning to see the picture appear. That was more than 30 years ago. Now, of course, none of what I've described above would be of any interest to any urban Chinese.

At that time only 800 privately owned cars navigated the streets of Beijing. The rest of the vehicles were either cabs or Chinese army vehicles— and, of course, some 6 million bicycles that moved like rivers of dark-blue-clad riders on both sides of all major streets. Today the streets of Chinese cities are packed with private automobiles ranging from compact to ultra luxury cars.

We finally reconnected with our official welcoming party and appointed hosts and spent two days touring Beijing in the more conventional way with official guides. The fourth day we began a 16-hour train trip north to Harbin. Since China was a classless society there were no third-class, second-class, or first-class accommodations on the train. But we could buy hard seats, soft seats, or bunks. Go figure.

We made arrangements for bunks. That gave the four of us a room on the train about the size of my old VW van. To get down from my top bunk, I had to grab a pipe, hang down and drop between the two lower bunks. To get up I had to do the opposite. The train made one midafternoon stop at the station in Shenyang, a large industrial city with its omnipresent pollution nearly hiding the factories that gave the city its reason for existence.

The purpose of the stop was not only to disgorge passengers and take on an equal number of new passengers, mostly Red Army soldiers, but also to take on food. The food was an open mound of mostly green vegetables about 4 feet high and 6 to 8 feet in diameter piled on the concrete of the station platform. While the disembarking passengers were getting off and new passengers were getting on, workers were loading the vegetables into the "cooking car" with what I would describe as coal shovels. As I watched them shovel our meals from the floor of the train station platform to the floor of the cooking car, I realized it would be easy for me to judge the insulin required as long as they didn't put any unknown sweet sauces on the vegetables. They didn't. They simply boiled the vegetables, added a little salt, put the meal in a little bowl and sold it to the passengers for a few Chinese *yuan*—about 5 cents American.

I developed a pattern of blood sugar control on that visit to China that became my habit for all my foreign travel that would follow. I didn't try to keep my blood sugar in my normal range of 80 to 110 mg/dl. My target was 120 to 140. It was an active decision on my part to trade tight control for a short time of looser control and a lower risk of low blood sugar episodes in an unfamiliar country.

That habit has served me well and I recommend it for foreign travel if you're staying in a foreign country for a week or less. If your stay is longer than that, as you get more comfortable with your surroundings you should begin to tighten up your control.

In China it was pretty easy to keep my blood sugar under control most of the time. Our meals consisted primarily of simple preparations of fish, beef, pork, and vegetables. The exception was official dinners. In China, as in every communist country I visited in the early and mid '80s, official meals were as lavish and extravagant as any buffet in a five-star American hotel today.

China in the 1980s, while professing to be a classless society, had two classes apparent to me. The lower economic class consisted of peasant farmers and workers and in the upper class were political officials and government leaders. They were separated by an opaque lifestyle wall that functioned like a one-way mirror. The political officials could, of course see through this wall and know how the rest of the Chinese were living. The lower economic class, however, could never really see past their daily lives and witness the opulence surrounding the political officials.

Our arrival in Harbin began the official part of the trip. As we checked into our hotel, we were handed an English translation of the 10 rules for staying at the hotel. The rules were so entertaining I still have a copy in my files. Here is a word-for-word quote of rule 7:

> **Rule 7**. Within the hotel, the following conduct is prohibited: Get drunk and create a disturbance, come to blows, gambling, go whoring, drug taking, dissemination of reactionary, obscene, and superstitious books, pictures of promiscuous drugs, pornographic devices, and other criminal activities."

We decided we could meet those rules and we sure didn't have any pictures of promiscuous drugs.

Our host, Chairman Wang, was very gracious. We had a number of official meetings that focused on dealing with winter conditions in northern cities. Some of the ideas were applicable to Anchorage, but not the system of organized hand-shoveling of snow from the streets by citizens. I was pretty sure that the people of Anchorage wouldn't agree to hand-shovel the snow from their street before going to work in the morning, as was done in Harbin.

One of the most memorable hours of the trip for me was a meeting Chairman Wang and I had in a small, dingy hotel room with stained carpet and limp, dirty drapes. It was just the two of us and one interpreter. After some discussion about city business, I changed the tenor of the conversation by telling him about what American kids in the '50s had been worried about and talked about in their preteen and early teen years. The chairman was about 25 years older than I and had been in a leadership position in China when I was a young kid.

I told him as kids in the '50s we worried about the atomic bomb, about Russia and China joining forces and attacking the United States, and about the coming ice age that our parents said was imminent. We, of course, really knew nothing about those issues any more than we knew anything about car engines and sex, which we also talked a lot about. In those days in Southern California, bomb shelters were sold in many shopping center parking lots and many swimming pool companies were shifting to the higher-demand bomb shelter installation.

I was so concerned about the coming ice age when I was 11 that I bought a pair of ice skates for 10 cents from a friend who was going to throw them away. Even though I lived in Southern California, if the ice age came I was going to be ready. Although the ice age issue was frequently discussed in our parents' circles, it never really got a lot of national media attention because, unlike today, nobody could figure out who to blame. Now that climatic discussion has shifted to the global warming end of the climatic spectrum it's getting a lot more attention because there are targets for the media to blame: the oil industry, the auto industry, and the coal industry.

What I talked to Chairman Wang about that day was not the ice age but the previous undercurrent of worry in the United States about Chinese aggression aimed toward us, especially in light of the Chinese role in the Korean War. Currently, aggression is no longer as big an issue as China's economic growth and competition with the United States, but at that time, Mao Tse-Tung had been dead only about six years and China was still very much under the influence of his policies.

Chairman Wang's response to me was very interesting. He said that China did not now have the political will, the economic strength, or the military capacity to even think about aggression against a power like the United States. I think we both felt quite free to talk openly since neither of us was in a decision-making position in the area of foreign policy. I thought a little about his interpreter reporting his statements to higher Communist party officials but he didn't seem worried about it.

More International Travel with Our Kids

Taking a Youth Baseball Team to Japan

It was about this time that we began more international travel with our kids. In the summer of 1983, after my trip to Japan with Mary and Rich, I made plans to take a group of 8- to 13-year-old neighborhood kids who had been on the Little League teams I had coached to Japan to compete against Japanese youth baseball teams. The logical choice for the visit and games was Chitose, Hokkaido in northern Japan. I coordinated the arrangements with the mayor of Chitose and the chairman of the Chitose assembly. I recruited my friend, Tim Rogers, to help organize the trip and help coach the team.

The trip was very positive in terms of our kids' understanding that youth from different cultures, who spoke in different languages, had the same feelings and expressions of excitement, fun, and laughter as the American kids had. Toward the end of the trip, we asked our youngsters if they thought we should invite the Japanese kids to Anchorage the following summer. They all thought we should and after some discussion with their parents upon our return home, we extended a reciprocal invitation to the Japanese kids and their coaches to come to Anchorage the next summer. The success and popularity of the exchange spread to other Alaskan youth baseball teams and the baseball exchanges between Alaska and Japan continued for many summers.

Venezuela and Peru

Shortly after we returned from Japan, Jenni, who was seven, declared that it was time for her to go on the next trip because "I'm already seven and I haven't even been to Japan yet." That perceived travel deficit on Jenni's part began changing a few years later when I took her with me on a trip to Venezuela and Peru along with Anne Arruda, an Olympic volunteer, interpreter, and all-around delightful travel advisor and assistant.

Anne was especially helpful when we had to change our flight from Venezuela to Peru via Bogotá, Colombia because the kids Jenni had met in Venezuela had told her that if we stopped in Colombia, she would be kidnapped and killed and her eyes would be removed and sold to hospitals there. Once stories like that get imbedded into a 10-year-old's mind, nothing can erase them. We had to get to Peru for some key Olympic meetings and the *only* option we had was to fly back to Miami, then reverse course and fly back to Lima, Peru.

Despite the very illogical route, it was going to work. The layover in Miami gave us enough time to change terminals and still make our nonstop flight to Lima in time for our meetings. Until the unexpected, and in my lifetime of travel, the unprecedented, happened. Avianca, the national airline of Venezuela, made an unscheduled and feebly explained landing at a remote island airport. None of the passengers on the plane seemed to know where we were. Anne was alternately talking to and yelling at the purser and the pilot explaining in the fastest Spanish I ever heard that we had a key connection to make in Miami in order to make our meeting in Peru. I'm not 100 percent sure but I thought I heard the name of the president of Peru, Alan Garcia Perez, being invoked in Anne's diatribe.

As Anne was verbally exploding at the pilot, I looked out the window and saw an old van pull up next to the plane. Two thirtyish-looking, shabbily dressed men jumped out and started catching small, identically wrapped packages being thrown out of the plane. They in turn threw the packages into the back of the van. After about three minutes and with maybe 60 packages having been transferred, the receivers jumped in the van and careened off the runway and disappeared down a dirt road. Now I don't know for sure what was in the packages but I'm pretty sure it wasn't Barbie dolls.

Anne had, unbelievably, gotten the pilot to agree to get our luggage out of the hold and put it in the passenger compartment. That action, as it would turn out, was crucial. When we got to Miami, I found a skycap, gave him a $50 bill and took out another $50 and told him it was his if we made our connection. With Jenni out in front, Anne carrying her purse and high heels, me waving a $50 bill and the skycap chasing us with our luggage on a cart, we made the quarter-mile sprint between terminals and made our connection to Lima.

Winter Trips to Austria, Switzerland, and Manchuria

A year later, Mary and I took all our kids on a ski trip to Innsbruck, Austria and Zermatt, Switzerland with our close friends, Dave and Peggy Baumeister and their three kids. Zermatt, a town at the base of the Matterhorn, is reachable only by cog rail and allows no private automobiles. After skiing all day, each evening we'd ski from our bed and breakfast hostel into the town for dinner. After dinner we loaded our skis on horse-drawn sleighs and clopped back up the hill to the hostel.

We also took our kids on a winter trip to the Manchuria area of northern China with our friends Eric Chan and Vicki Sun-Chan as our guides and interpreters. One of the most durable memories of that trip was taking a short—50 kilometers or so—trip from Harbin to the small city of Ah Cheng. The Mongolian desert landscape was white with a slight covering of snow, just enough to make the two-lane dirt road disappear into the whiteness. But it was no problem knowing where the road was. It was defined by long, continuous lines of expressionless peasants on both sides of the road, each pulling a handcart loaded with goods being moved between the two cities. They were all dressed in heavy, warm-looking, dark jackets and pants that served as both their working and sleeping clothes.

Our interpreter explained that each one-way segment took one day and that the cart-pullers would make three round trips a week. While they were at their destination city, they would pay the equivalent of five American cents for soup, rice, and a floor to sleep on. The next day they would return to their home city. This they would do six days a week with the seventh day off.

By the time we got to Ah Cheng, we were hungry and feeling a little guilty about it after watching all the people pulling the carts and only getting rice and soup at the end of their journey. But the meal the mayor of Ah Cheng had prepared was modest enough to assuage our guilt. It was one big, catfish-looking monster on the center of the table and what looked like baby chicks that had been fried whole in sizzling grease. Mary and I ate enough to be polite and the kids ate peanut butter and crackers that Mary had been smart enough to stuff in her suitcase before we left Alaska. We also found that in that part of China, even the people who work inside wore their full winter coats all day long since the inside temperature of the buildings was barely kept above freezing. In fact, to wash our hands in the wash bowl in the city building at Ah Cheng, we had to break the thin layer of ice in the wash bowl with our fingers.

Time Zone Changes and Blood Sugar Control

Whether you use a pump or not, you can adapt to major time zone changes without blood sugar control problems. One key is to not change your watch when you leave your departure city. Insulin is being absorbed by your body based on your departure city time zone, so keep it that way until about three to four hours after you've arrived at your destination. This will give you a chance to see how tired you are and what your eating schedule will be, and to estimate how long it may take to get on your new time zone schedule.

In general, if you are traveling west, for example to Asia, or east to west across the United States, you will be very tired when you arrive and will find it hard to stay awake past eight or nine o'clock in the evening. The good thing about westward travel is that you'll be in bed early the first night and up early the next day. Eastward travel is more difficult because you'll find yourself lying awake at night and being very tired in the morning. Eastward travel makes it harder to adapt your sleeping schedule as well as your blood sugar control.

Introducing Our Kids to the Rest of America

Mystrom Advertising had grown to about 45 very committed and competent employees under the leadership of our department heads Dennis Smith, Marsha Wilson, Cheri Gillian, Wanda Galyan, Hilary Hilscher, and soon-to-be vice president Linda Boochever. I had purchased a downtown office with Mystrom Advertising as the primary tenant and in a moment of generous exuberance, I bought new Volvos for all our account executives to use.

Our kids were doing well in school, taking part in school activities, playing sports year-round and leading fun-filled, active, healthy lives. We were blessed that Mary was able to be a full-time mom except for a couple of years when we first moved to Alaska and had little money. For a couple of years she worked as an office supply salesperson, and then part of a summer as a compactor (we used to call them steamrollers) operator for Uchitel Construction.

About that time Mary and I started a series of family vacations that I would recommend to any American family with young kids. Because we live in Alaska, we had done most of our Lower 48 travel only to California to visit my relatives, to Wisconsin to visit Mary's relatives, and to Hawaii for our family vacations. We recognized that our kids had really seen little of America at ground level.

The kids now ranged in age from 6 to 10, so we decided that over the next five years we would introduce them to our wonderful country. We divided the United States into five regions: the west coast, the Rocky Mountain west, mid-America, the southeast, and the northeast. Our plan was to fly to a starting point, rent a car and begin a weeklong, leisurely tour through that area of America. The trip would end with another week at a "reward destination" so we always had a destination for the kids to anticipate. The reward destinations were Disneyland in California, a ranch in Colorado, a cabin and houseboat on Lake Geneva in Wisconsin, and Disneyworld in Florida.

What made the trips so successful was that we didn't start too early each morning and we never drove for more than about four or five hours a day. We'd visit all the fun places along the way, especially water parks, and we'd stop early enough in the afternoon to enjoy family swims at a motel with a swimming pool. They weren't exactly cultural immersion experiences but they were fun and bonding. One of everyone's favorite segments was concluding the mid-America trip by taking the American Eagle Amtrak train from Chicago to Dallas. It was a 24-hour trip that was so much fun that none of us wanted it to end. A train trip through America presents a snapshot of America's backyard—a Norman-Rockwell-meets-Ansel-Adams landscape of America.

A year after our mid-America trip, I took our two boys and two friends back to the Drowsy Water Ranch in Colorado for a repeat week. The boys and their friends, Alonzo and Ted, were 12 and 14 years old and enjoyed the all-guys' vacation.

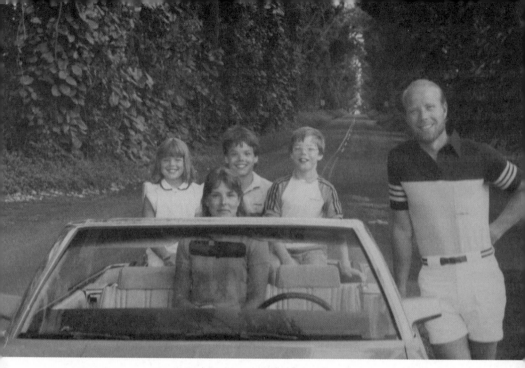

Our family on one of our trips to discover America.

Working at the ranch for the summer were more than a dozen college kids, about half of them guys and half girls. The guys were all football players from the University of Utah, men physically, but not emotionally or mentally, had been throwing the girls in a scudsy pond that separated the horse corral from the main ranch house. The girls were trying to figure out a way to throw the guys in the pond but they were just too strong.

They asked us to help throw the guys in. But adding a 40-year-old man, two 14-year-olds and two 12-year-olds to the girls' side wasn't going to work against eight big and athletic 20-year-old studs. But I offered an idea to the girls and they loved it. So at dinner that night I challenged the football players from Utah to a volleyball game. They would pick their best two athletes to play a volleyball game against me and my 14-year-old, 5-foot-9, 120-pound son, Nick. If they won they could throw us in the pond. If we won, the girls could throw them in the pond.

I told them what wimps they would be if they didn't accept the challenge of a 40-year-old man, 10 years past his prime, and a 14-year-old boy, 10 years away from his prime. Sometimes stories get softened in memoirs and this might be one because I'm pretty sure I didn't use the word *wimps*.

Well, they accepted the challenge. They had to. Nick and I killed them in the volleyball game but the guys didn't exactly let the girls throw them in. As soon as we finished them off in two straight games, they all ran straight to the scum pond and dove in. Not exactly the bet but good enough to give the girls the satisfaction they wanted.

To this day, we talk about the enjoyment we had as a family on those trips. When that four-year experience ended—we actually never did the northeast—we felt that the kids had at least an introduction to America.

Travel whenever you're able to. Don't ever let diabetes keep you from the wonderful experiences and future heartfelt memories that travel provides. As children, my sisters and I loved our annual two-week trips from Pennsylvania to Minnesota and as adults Mary and I and our kids have enjoyed and learned from our travels around the world.

During that period, we had a little adventure at home that made the front page of one of our papers. It was about midnight on Friday night. Nick was 14, Rich was 12, and Jenni was 9. Mary and I were in bed when Nick opened our bedroom door and said, "Dad?" I sat up and said, "What?" Nick said, "You're here! Then someone's stealing our car. Right now. They're trying to start it." I jumped out of bed and ran down the stairs in my underwear. Nick was right behind me, Mary behind him, and Rich following with Jenni coming too.

It's amazing how much goes through one's mind when adrenaline is pumping. If I went out the side garage door, I could surprise him. I'd go for the driver's door and jump in. As I sprinted out the door, I thought I saw two people in the car. The car was out on the street but the thief couldn't keep it running.

I yelled to Nick to take the passenger, I'd get the driver. Not knowing if he had a weapon, I knew I'd have to immobilize his hands. I'd grab his left wrist with my left hand, grab his neck with my right hand and pile in on top of him. All of this went through my mind in about three seconds. It worked perfectly except that Nick wasn't behind me. He had stopped to get a baseball bat out of the trash can that held sports gear.

I dove into the car. And it worked exactly as I planned. I was on top of the driver holding his wrist with my left hand and his neck with my right hand. The "passenger" turned out to be a backpack he had stolen from our other car. I yelled to Nick to call 911, then turned to see him holding the baseball bat and sounding like the 14-year-old he was. "Hey dude, we've got you now. You picked the wrong family, dude." I told him to stay where he was and yelled to Mary to call 911.

The cops got there in about two minutes and took over. As I told the newspaper reporter who called the next day, "After it was over we all went inside, woke up our watchdog, Heidi, and told and retold the story for about an hour."

The next five years would require more travel to more foreign countries than I could have ever anticipated. That worldwide travel was triggered by a simple question I asked myself as I watched the television coverage of the Winter Olympic Games in Sarajevo, Yugoslavia. The question was: Why can't Alaska host the Winter Olympics?

Ask not alone for victory but ask for courage. For if you endure, you bring honor to yourself. Even more you bring honor to us all.

—Charge given to the ancient Olympians as they entered the arena

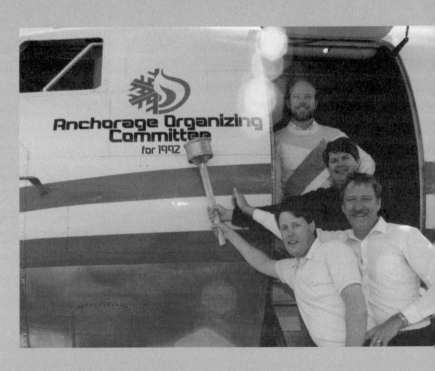

Leaders of the Anchorage Organizing Committee just prior to boarding the chartered plane for presentation to the USOC in Indianapolis. *Front to back:* Rick Nerland, Bob Penney, Dick Angell, and I.

Chapter 10

Alaska's Olympic Dreams

My Long Fascination with the Olympics

In 1952, when I was an eight-year-old in Lewisburg, Pennsylvania, my exposure to sports news was limited to *Movietone News* at the Campus or Roxy theaters, *Boys' Life* magazine, *Reader's Digest* and *Life* magazines, and most influential of all, the back of Wheaties boxes.

We did have a big wooden radio which stood on our living room floor and towered above me. My sisters, Rosanne, who was 10, and Rochelle, who was six, and I would sit on the floor and stare up at the big round illuminated dial. We were fascinated by the detective work of Mr. and Mrs. North. We loved comparing Ozzie and Harriet to our family, and we'd laugh in anticipation every time Fibber Magee opened his closet door and released a clattering avalanche of junk.

But I was the only one of the kids who listened to sports and the only sports that earned a locked-in spot in my memory 60 years later were the New York Yankees games against my favorite team, the Brooklyn Dodgers, in the 1952 and 1953 World Series. My friends and I bet on the games. A nickel was the highest stake I remember.

The Dodgers lost both of those World Series but during one of them my dad gave me some advice I've never forgotten. He said, "Son, you can cheer for the Dodgers but bet on the Yankees." In broader terms he was saying, "Don't let your emotions influence your investments." That bit of philosophy has served me well in investments and real estate purchases throughout my life.

We, of course, had no television at that time. It was 30 years later that I told my then five-year-old son, Richard, that we didn't get a television set until I was 12. He pondered the statement for a moment, then said, "Dad, if you didn't have a television set, how did you watch TV?"

In the year 1952 Bob Mathias won his second gold medal in the decathlon at the Olympic Games in Helsinki. His first was in London in 1948, the first Olympics held since the propaganda-laced 1936 Olympics in Berlin orchestrated by Adolf Hitler. Bob Mathias was everywhere in the sports news in my world but it was the front and back of the Wheaties boxes that I read every morning over my big bowl of Wheaties, "breakfast of champions." I was absolutely sure that someplace in America Bob Mathias was eating his Wheaties with sliced bananas just like I was.

As I grew, my interest in the Olympics grew also. The names still stick in my mind: Bobby Murrow, the great American sprinter and triple gold medalist in the '56 games in Melbourne, Muhammad Ali (then Cassius Clay) winning the light-heavyweight gold in Rome in 1960. And in 1964 in Tokyo, the expected 100-meter win of the world's fastest man, Bob Hayes, and the totally unexpected win of the unknown American, Billy Mills, a Lakota Sioux, in the 10,000 meter race.

But it was Bob Beamon in the 1968 Olympics in Mexico City who provided the single most memorable Summer Olympic moment in my lifetime: at that time the world record for the long jump was 27 feet 4¾ inches. Journalists speculated about when or if the seemingly improbable 28-foot mark would be reached. Bob Beamon not only reached the 28-foot mark but he passed it in the air and didn't come down until he had also passed the 29-foot mark. His jump of 29 feet 2⅜ inches was so far beyond human capabilities at that time that no one, including Bob Beamon, even reached 28 feet for a decade after "the Leap." In fact, Beamon was booed on a tour of Europe right after the Mexico City Olympics because he jumped only about 27 feet in exhibitions.

Four years before "the leap of the century," the Winter Olympics (officially the Olympic Winter Games) began capturing my attention. Two schoolmates of mine at the University of Colorado, Billy Kidd and Jimmy Huega, won silver and bronze in the Innsbruck Olympic Winter Games in 1964.

Then in the 1968 Winter Olympics in Grenoble, France's Jean Claude Killy captured the attention of the sporting world by sweeping all the alpine skiing events with gold medals in the downhill, the giant slalom, and the slalom. Eighteen years later, I found myself competing against Killy in a different Olympic arena. We were each representing our respective countries in their bids to host the 1992 Olympic Winter Games—he was the honorary chairman of France's bid and I was the chairman of America's bid.

In the 1976 Olympic Winter Games in Innsbruck, Austria, the great downhill run of the Austrian Franz Klammer was the defining moment; it is still considered the best downhill run in Olympic history.

Denver's Bid for the Olympic Winter Games

The right to host the 1976 Olympic Winter Games had been won by Denver, Colorado but based on a statewide referendum in November 1972 that opposed Denver hosting the games, Denver officially withdrew their bid on November 15. With less than 15 months before opening ceremonies were scheduled to begin, the Winter Olympics had no host city and were in danger of being canceled for the first time since World War II.

But Innsbruck, Austria stepped forward. They had hosted the Winter Olympics in 1964. The medium-sized alpine city had the facilities in place and its citizens had both the desire and the ability to make the games happen in less than 15 months. Thirty-seven nations took part in the opening ceremonies on February 4, 1976 and the Olympic Games' peacetime continuity remained unbroken.

The bitter taste of that rejection still remains within the collective memory of the International Olympic Committee. In the late 1980s, I had a number of conversations with members of the IOC who said that if Denver were the only city competing to host the Olympic Winter Games, they would cancel the games rather than give them to Denver. I expect the bad feelings have faded slightly since then but it is certainly a barrier that Denver would have to deal with if it ever chose to bid again.

The Miracle on Ice

In 1980 at the Lake Placid Olympic Winter Games came "the miracle on ice," one of the greatest and most improbable sporting upsets of all time. A collection of American college kids, amateurs all, faced off against the pride of the USSR, the Red Army team, in the semifinals.

The game was set during the height of the Cold War, with ongoing tension between the two great superpowers, the United States and the Soviet Union. For years we had used the free and prosperous lives of our citizens as evidence of the superiority of our system of government and the Soviet Union under Premier Brezhnev countered with the health and athletic superiority of its citizens as evidence of the superiority of their system. And nowhere did the Soviets attempt to display their citizens' health and athletic dominance more convincingly than in the Olympic Games.

For 20 years leading up to the 1980 Olympic Winter Games in Lake Placid, the Soviet Union had dominated many Olympic sports. The hockey dominance of the USSR was almost absolute. They had lost only one of the 30 games in Olympic hockey competition since the 1960 Olympic Winter Games in Squaw Valley. In the year leading up to the 1980 Winter Games, they had embarrassed a National Hockey League all-star team, made up of the best professional hockey players in the free world, by a score of 6–0. That would be comparable to 42–0 in a football game.

It was David vs. Goliath, Mike Tyson vs. Buster Douglas, Tiger Woods vs. Tony the Tiger. The Soviet Union was certain to continue its dominance and add evidence to the claims that its political system produced physical superiority. How could this team of college kids led by a college coach, Herb Brooks of the University of Minnesota, even claim they belonged on the same ice as the pride of the Soviet Union?

Well, they belonged. The US team faced the Soviet Union in a semifinal match. At the end of the first period the game was tied 2–2. By the end of the second period, the US team was down by only one point,

3–2. Unbelievably, the American team scored twice in the last period. The last goal came with 10 minutes left in the game and the United States took its first lead in the game, 4–3. For the last 10 minutes the American-dominated crowd stood and screamed together as did millions of American families watching it on television. With 10 seconds left the frenzied crowd began counting down. TV announcer Al Michaels began his now famous call, "You've got ten seconds left, the countdown going on right now… five seconds left in the game. DO YOU BELIEVE IN MIRACLES? YES!"

For the International Hockey Federation it was the hockey story of the century. For America it was simply "the miracle on ice."

The Seeds of Anchorage's Bid for the Winter Olympics

At the Conference of Northern Mayors in Sapporo, Japan that I had attended at the request of Mayor Knowles, the mayor of Sapporo spoke glowingly about how Sapporo's hosting of the Winter Olympics in 1972 had improved their city. He said people around the world knew Sapporo primarily because it had been an Olympic city. He said that the economy in general, and tourism in specific, experienced major and continuing improvement as a result of hosting the Winter Olympics. But most important, he said, was their citizens' more positive attitude toward their city.

Sapporo's experiences were consistent with what I had concluded from media coverage of past games. Olympics hosting and participation seemed to enhance national, state, and city pride and also seemed to promote international good-will. It was with this mindset that I began reading, with a different perspective, the articles leading up to the February, 1984 Olympic Winter Games in Sarajevo, Yugoslavia.

At that time, I was chairman of the Anchorage Assembly and I started thinking about Anchorage hosting the Olympic Winter Games. I began asking myself questions. How does a city get the Olympic Games? Is it the country that gets them first and then chooses the city? Or does a country first choose a city to represent the country? Who makes the decisions? Who pays for the games? Who gets the revenues?

Then the real question in my mind: *Could Anchorage host the Winter Olympics?*

Honestly, I didn't know the answers to any of those questions. But I knew one person who might, Chris Von Imhof. Chris was the very well known and well-liked manager of the Alyeska Ski Resort, Alaska's major ski area. He was born in Garmisch-Partenkirchen, Germany, host city of the 1936 Olympic Winter Games. Chris was born after those Olympic Games but he grew up in an Olympic city and he spoke with a German accent. That made him the closest thing to an expert that I could conjure up. Plus he was one of the most positive, can-do people I knew. So I called him.

Chris and I met for lunch that week at the Corsair restaurant in Anchorage. Up to that point, most of the people I had talked to about the idea had been politely skeptical: "We're too small." "Too isolated." "Too cold." "Too dark." "Not enough snow." "Too much snow." "Too few hotel rooms." "Too few winter competition facilities." "Nobody will come." It will be a failure." "Too many people will come. It will be too crowded." Some were not so polite: "A bonehead idea. A waste of money. You're nuts." And my favorite: "If it doesn't snow, we'll ruin our reputation." My question was "What reputation?" At that time more tourists went to Death Valley in midsummer than came to Alaska in midwinter.

But Chris was different. Not only did he think we could do it but he committed to doing everything he could to help lead the effort. Chris also added quite a bit to my modest store of information on the selection process and requirements to host the games. Along with his unconditional support, he also added great connection to the Alaska visitor industry. I left that meeting ready to act.

Organizing Anchorage's Bid Committee

I started by recruiting friends and acquaintances in the Anchorage business and sports communities to serve on a steering committee. This committee would go through the process of setting up a board of directors; then the committee would dissolve and the board would take over. By late March 1984, we had a steering committee of 12 people. According to newspaper articles, the steering committee included a number of business leaders who would become leaders of our bid. In addition to Chris, they included Dave Baumeister, president of an aviation company and one of the most quietly competent people I have ever known. Dave had just returned from the Olympic Winter Games in Sarajevo and was one of the first people to step up and commit to helping lead the bid. Others were Chris Swalling, a highly regarded CPA committed to community and family; Carl Brady, an insurance company owner and community leader; Bob Hickel, an operator of

family-owned shopping malls throughout Alaska; Peter Lekisch, a successful attorney and endurance athlete; Max Nalley, a bright and competent Exxon executive; Al Parrish, a hotelier and business leader; Bob Penney, a successful entrepreneur, community leader, and source of boundless energy and ideas; and former Anchorage mayor George Sullivan. We gathered information about the

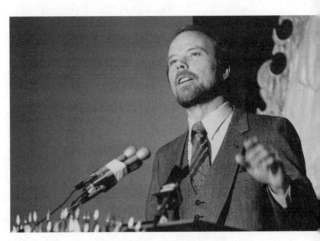

My first speech introducing the idea of Anchorage hosting the Winter Olympics, given to Anchorage Downtown Rotary, April 3, 1984.

process of bidding, communicated our interest to the United States Olympic Committee, and began discussing the possibility of hosting the games.

In early February, 1984, the *Anchorage Times* wrote the first article about what we were considering. They followed it up with a positive editorial a few days later. On April 3 I made my first speech on the possibility of hosting the Olympic Winter Games to the Downtown Rotary Club.

The outline of the speech was simple and so effective that it became the basis of over 100 speeches I would give in Alaska and around the world over the next five years supporting Anchorage's bid for the Olympic Winter Games. I asked and answered three questions: "Should we host the Olympic Winter Games?" "Can we host the Winter Games?" and "How do we do it?"

Some of the questions from skeptics were easy to answer in my speech:

Too isolated? No. Not unless you think of St. Louis, Missouri as the center of the world. If that were the case then we'd be in the upper left hand corner of the world. But from an international perspective, Anchorage is very central. With over 100 international flights a week in and out of Anchorage in 1984, we were nine hours nonstop to Frankfurt, eight hours to London, and just over seven hours to Seoul and Tokyo. As I said in my speeches, "Anchorage is equidistant from the population centers of North America, Europe, and Asia."

Too small? Heck no. At that time we would have been the fourth-largest city to ever host the Olympic Winter Games. Only Oslo, Sapporo, and Sarajevo were larger.

Not enough hotel rooms, too few spectators? I thought then and confirmed later that the International Olympic Committee and the United States Olympic Committee would be more interested in Anchorage's perfect time zone for the United States TV market than they were in the number of live spectators who would attend the games. As one IOC member later said to me: "We care less about the fact that your hockey arena seats only 6,000 than we do about the additional 60 million people who will watch the Winter Olympics live on American TV." An event final held in Anchorage at 4 p.m. would air at 8 p.m. in New York, 7 p.m. in Chicago, 6 p.m. in Denver, and 5 p.m. in Los Angeles—prime time across America. The American TV market was then and is now the dominant funding source for both the Summer and the Winter Olympic Games.

Another question was tougher to answer: *Can we do it with private funding?* I didn't know. But Los Angeles, with the IOC's approval, was attempting to host a privately funded Olympic Games that summer and we would find out if it could be done.

The Downtown Rotary speech ended with a standing ovation from the overflow crowd. After some time for questions, the meeting ended with lines of people wanting to sign up to volunteer. The speech was a front-page story in both daily newspapers and was followed by positive editorials in both papers a few days later. That speech on April 3, 1984 marked the beginning of Anchorage's five-year quest to host the Olympic Winter Games and the beginning of my five-year commitment as the volunteer leader of the bid.

With input from Chris Von Imhof and other business leaders, we put together a Bid Committee. The Anchorage Organizing Committee for the Winter Olympics was shortened to just the "Anchorage Organizing Committee," then referred to as the AOC. I was elected president and Chris Swalling was elected vice president. Later, I would become chairman and Dave Baumeister would be elected president and Chris would be vice president and treasurer. We formed an executive committee made up of the early business leaders I had recruited plus Bill Tobin, managing editor of the *Anchorage Times*; Linda Chase, a dynamic and creative Anchorage businesswoman; Dick Angell, a banker and a bit of a wheeler-dealer; and Tony Smith, a bright and garrulous attorney.

The Deadline That Energized Anchorage

We made slow, steady progress for six to seven months, learning what we could and developing strategies, but in March, 1985, everything changed. We got a call from the United States Olympic Committee saying that they had decided to sponsor a candidate city for the Olympic Winter Games of 1992 and asked if we wanted to compete against Salt Lake City, Lake Placid, and Reno-Tahoe for the right to be America's candidate.

The competition would be held on June 15, 1985 in Indianapolis at the annual meeting of the United States Olympic Committee. We would have one half hour to make our presentation. We would also be expected to prepare brochures, technical booklets, and an exhibit to support our bid. We committed to being a candidate within days.

We had the organization in place and just a month earlier had made what turned out to be an extraordinarily good decision. We hired Rick Nerland as executive director of our bid. Rick had been the vice president of the family-owned Nerland's Home Furnishing, Alaska's largest and oldest furniture retailer. At only 33 years old, he was an excellent organizer, not intimidated by any challenge or any person. He was well connected to the business and athletic community in Anchorage and he was well-organized and goal-oriented, a perfect choice.

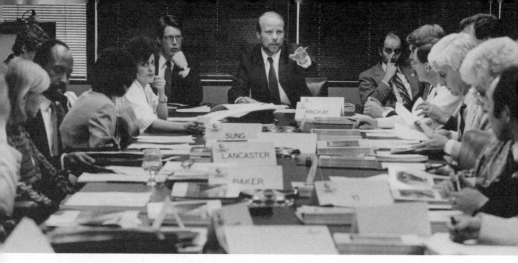

An Anchorage Organizing Committee board meeting after selection as America's candidate for the 1992 Olympic Winter Games. By that time I was chairman, Dave Baumeister, to my left, was president, and Rick Nerland, to my right, was executive director.

Photo courtesy of Anchorage Daily News

Our task was clear. We had three months to determine the location of all the different competition sites and venues; to write, design, and produce both technical and promotional booklets and brochures; to conceive, design, and produce from scratch a dramatic, persuasive exhibit that we could tear down and rebuild in Indianapolis; and to write a convincing and compelling presentation supported by the technology of the day, a multi-projector slideshow—and we had to raise the money to do all that.

It never occurred to any of the AOC leadership or volunteers that we couldn't do all that in three months. And, as in other challenges in my life, it never occurred to me that diabetes would have any hindering impact on my ability to provide the leadership to make a successful bid.

I would be writing the presentation and delivering it on behalf of Anchorage. What did enter my mind a number of times over the next three months was that I didn't want to have, or even be concerned about having, low blood sugar during the presentation. The solution was pretty simple. I would test my blood sugar twice before my presentation: once an hour before and once more about 10 minutes before to see where my blood sugar was and what direction it was headed. My goal was to be between 150 and

200, which is high under normal conditions but would provide a comfortable margin of protection against low blood sugar in the high-pressure, inflexible situation I'd be experiencing. As a further backup I would keep a glass of Seven-Up at the podium instead of the standard glass of water.

As it would turn out, through five years of world travel and scores of speeches on behalf of Anchorage and the United States Olympic Committee, I never did have any extreme low blood sugars related directly to the bid activity.

With Dave Baumeister and Rick Nerland assembling the technical data and organizing the volunteers, Linda Chase creating and organizing the exhibits, Bob Penney, Carl Brady, Bob Hickel, and Ed Rasmuson, president of National Bank of Alaska raising the money we needed, I was free to generate support for the bid from the U.S. Olympic Committee, from the citizens of Anchorage, and from the rest of Alaska.

In addition to building support among Alaskans, I was working with the talented and committed Mystrom Advertising employees to prepare the presentation for the USOC. My goal was to complete it in two months and have time to rehearse and fine-tune it in front of the AOC Executive Committee, then make the presentation in front of the Chamber of Commerce, the Anchorage Downtown and the Anchorage East Rotary Clubs, which I hoped would get the positive publicity necessary to strengthen the commitment of the Alaskan public.

It was an exciting, energy-filled three months and we met all our goals. Before the deadline set by the USOC, we had been making slow and somewhat unsteady progress. But the deadline changed everything. We *had* to put it all together by the deadline and we did. By the time the deadline arrived, we were ready. The technical manual was done. The exhibits were completed, the presentation was done, and a beautiful brochure touting Anchorage as a site was produced.

Presentation rehearsals to the Chamber and the Rotary Clubs were met with enthusiastic standing ovations. To further develop interest, excitement, and support among Alaskans statewide, I also did a final presentation rehearsal in front of a standing-room-only crowd at our 2,500-seat Egan Convention Center with statewide TV coverage throughout Alaska.

Everyone on our committee was confident and the people of Anchorage were supportive but I kind of felt that many were preparing to say, "Nice try, good effort, you did the best you could," when we returned after not winning. Fortunately, no one would ever have to offer those kinds of sympathetic condolences.

The importance of a deadline in energizing any group toward a goal cannot be underestimated. Almost 20 years later, as a founding board member of the Alaska Sports Hall of Fame, I saw the same thing happening: a group of young, hard-working, smart people were trying to start the organization and create a selection process. After months of slow and intermittent progress, I related the story of our Olympic bid to them. I suggested that the best thing we could do right then was to pick a date for the first induction, make that date public and then figure out the details. We did exactly that and six months later we had our first Alaska Sports Hall of Fame induction ceremony. We're now coming up on our eighth annual ceremony, each one a highlight for the sports community in Alaska.

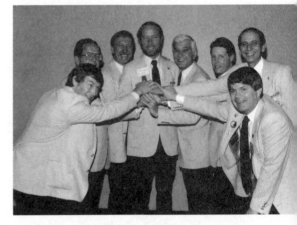

The Presentation to the USOC

At midnight on June 12, 1985, some 35 volunteers and a handful of staff members took off for Indianapolis on a plane pro-

Part of the AOC leadership team just prior to the winning presentation to the USOC. *Left to right:* Chris Swalling, Senator Ted Stevens, Bob Penney, me, Max Nalley, Rick Nerland, Dave Baumeister, and Dick Angell.

vided free to the committee by ERA Aviation. It was a propeller-driven Convair 550, its cargo hold loaded with our exhibits, brochures, presentation equipment, *and* a 60-pound king salmon caught two days earlier by Bob Penney.

The Convair rumbled along at about 340 miles per hour. We had to stop to refuel in Seattle and again in Grand Island, Nebraska, not exactly a metropolitan airport with a selection of restaurants. The trip was somewhere between 10 hours and forever. I can't exactly recall.

We arrived midafternoon on the 13th and got to work. On the day of the presentation all four competing cities had exhibits set up in the Indiana Convention Center and were making final preparations for their presentations before the USOC. All four of the competing cities had their own strengths and weaknesses:

Lake Placid, as the host of both the 1932 and 1980 Winter Olympics had many of the facilities already in place. As it turned out, having the facilities was also one of their weaknesses. The USOC and most of the National Governing Bodies (NGBs) would rather see the games at sites that would have to build new competition facilities. Another strength that Lake Placid talked about was the strong support that the federal government, the New York state government and the New York City municipal government and financial community had all brought to the table for the 1980 games. Lake Placid also projected the greatest surplus in its financial presentation.

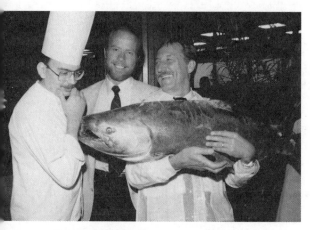

Bob Penney presents a 60-pound Alaska king salmon for a buffet hosted by the AOC in Indianapolis.

Reno-Tahoe touted their well-known ski areas in the indisputably beautiful setting surrounding Lake Tahoe. They also stated that the 14 million people in nearby northern California, at an easy driving distance from Reno-Tahoe, would result in "… one of the best attended Olympics of all time" according to their spokesman, Bill Martin. He said that organized gambling would also be an attractor, though some looked at that as a potential bid killer.

Salt Lake City promoted the advantages of being a large metropolitan area with well-developed and well-known ski resorts. I smiled at the comment of Tom Welch, the leader of the Salt Lake bid, who said, "We think we have even better air connections than Anchorage and we have the arts." Take that, Anchorage. The Salt Lake City Organizing Committee under Tom Welch later faced allegations of bribing both USOC and IOC members. The investigations following those allegations triggered a major reorganizing of the USOC and the resignations of a number of IOC members.

Even though Salt Lake City had excellent alpine ski resorts and even though alpine skiing was most often the focus of media coverage, a number of other winter sports had large followings and strong support groups within the Olympic movement. At that time hockey, figure skating, speed skating, biathlon, bobsled, and luge all had their own governing bodies, whereas all the skiing events were represented by the United States Ski Association, and all had a say in the decision to select an American candidate for the 1992 Olympic Winter Games. Salt Lake City's altitude, which we perceived as a problem for the aerobically challenging cross-country and biathlon events, and their disproportionate emphasis on alpine skiing seemed to us to be their only weaknesses.

I watched Salt Lake City technicians in matching uniforms set up their 15-projector slide show as our single technician, Bruce Graham, a skinny young guy in Levis and a T-shirt looked for a three-pronged adapter for our three-projector slide show. My mind flashed back to the Brooklyn Dodgers facing the New York Yankees in the 1955 World Series; Joe Namath and the New York Jets facing Johnny Unitas and the Baltimore Colts in Super Bowl III; and the US hockey team facing the Soviet Union in the 1980 Winter Olympics. They all won. So could we. I really believed.

The City of Anchorage is a young city by American standards: just 70 years old then. The Municipality of Anchorage, a merger of the old city government and the borough (county) government, was only 10 years old and in a lot of ways our city was like a fast-growing teenager: a little gangly and uncoordinated. We had had zoning for only about 20 years. Before that everything was built wherever anybody wanted. No rules. So it's fair to say we had a few blemishes. But we had some significant advantages and I knew these had to come across clearly and concisely in the presentation. If I could do that and then have the USOC members feel the emotion, excitement, and support of our citizens, we could win the bid.

Alaska's senior senator, Ted Stevens, led off our presentation and touched on his leadership in creating the Amateur Sports Act of 1978, which established the structure of the USOC and national governing bodies for individual sports. In other words, "You're here now when we need you because I was there then when you needed me." Well, he didn't exactly say it that way but it was out there. Other cities had governors or mayors to kick off their presentation and introduce their presenters, but we had "Uncle Ted."

After about five minutes, the senator introduced me. My blood sugar was right where I wanted it to be: 180. I had measured about an hour earlier and it was 190. It was going down slowly; that meant I had some insulin going into my body. Normally, if my blood sugar was 180, I'd give myself 1.6 units of insulin to bring it down to about 100 but in a competitive or pressure situation I burned more calories, which would lower my blood sugar faster than normal. So I left my blood sugar right there at 180 and took any worries about low blood sugar out of my mind.

I guess you could call that a pressure situation. On the line was a billion-dollar franchise for our city, a once-in-a-lifetime chance for our young people to see the Winter Olympics in person, a life-enriching experience for all our people and a historic event that would be part of Alaskans' collective memory for generations, and part of its history forever.

I didn't think about all that. I did think that the presentation could be very logically persuasive and very emotionally moving but a flawless delivery would be necessary to carry it off.

I started by recognizing that the Olympic Winter Games would bring much to our city—international recognition, a legacy of facilities and experiences, a bountiful sense of community pride, and a deeper sense of international understanding.

I talked about the issues that I knew would be brought up by skeptics:

Our location — Less than nine hours nonstop from northern Europe and northern Asia and a perfect location for liveTV for the American market. A 4 p.m. final in Anchorage would be 8 p.m. in New York, 7 p.m. in Chicago, 6 p.m. in Denver and 5 p.m. in Los Angeles—prime time across America.

Our access — Daily airline lift capacity at that time was 11,000 passengers per day in and out of Anchorage.

Our daylight — Anchorage had 21 minutes more daylight in February than the average of all previous Olympic Winter Games.

Our temperature — Over the past 40 years, our average February temperature had been 17.7 degrees Fahrenheit—perfect for winter sports.

Our snowfall — Over the past 39 years our average annual snowfall had been 69 inches with 12.3 inches of new snow in February.

Our facilities — We had good core facilities for Nordic skiing, biathlon, figure skating, and hockey. In fact, of the five Olympic-size hockey rinks in America at that time three were in or near Anchorage. We had a great mountain for the alpine events but we would need to build more base facilities. We would have to construct facilities for ski jumping, speed skating, and opening ceremonies. Fairbanks, our neighbor city to the north already had a recreational bob and luge course and was interested in building an Olympic-quality competition venue and wanted to be the site of the bob and luge competition. Working with the University of Alaska, we would construct the athletes' village, which would become dormitories for the University of Alaska, Anchorage after the games.

Throughout my presentation, we highlighted the beauty and mystical appeal of Alaska, the enthusiasm and strong, committed support of our people and the can-do frontier spirit that epitomizes our state.

I concluded my presentation to the USOC with these words:

> Today, you speak for America!
>
> Your choice is difficult but your responsibility is clear: To choose the city that represents our nation's best opportunity to return the Olympics to America.
>
> That city is Anchorage, Alaska. A vibrant, young, international city, accessible to the world, in a beautiful setting, with an ideal climate. A city filled with energy, excited by the challenge, united by the Olympic spirit, and committed to bringing the Olympic Winter Games back to America.

The response was far greater than we could have ever hoped. I think our whole committee sensed the rapture of the audience, their fascination with Alaska, and their apparent enthusiasm at the conclusion that Anchorage could actually do this.

Two hours later in a large room filled with all the candidate cities' contingents and members of the national press, Bob Helmick, president of the USOC, announced their decision with these words: "The United States Olympic Committee will be sponsoring the bid of *Anchorage*."

Those words set off a wild celebration from the Anchorage group who broke into spontaneous, enthusiastic rendition of our city's song, "Wild About Anchorage." Now that was years before Al Gore invented the Internet and the word back to Anchorage was not instantaneous. Rosemary Shinohara, a reporter at the *Anchorage Daily News*, told me later that the news of Anchorage's victory came over the teletype. She saw it first and yelled it out to the newsroom, "Anchorage won." Some laughed because they thought she was joking.

Within 10 minutes, members of our group were lined up at pay phones calling the newspapers, radio stations, and TV stations in Alaska. The most common reactions were "Really?" "Wow!" "No kidding!"

Anchorage's radio stations broke into their programming to make the announcement and all the TV stations pulled other stories and led their evening news with the story.

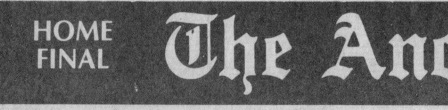

HOME FINAL · **The An**

ALASKA'S LARGEST NEWSPAPER/71st year   SUNDAY MO

ANCHOR

Banner headline in the *Anchorage Times* announces the result of
our competition with Salt Lake City, Reno-Tahoe, and Lake Placid
for the right to become America's candidate for the 1992 Olympic
Winter Games.

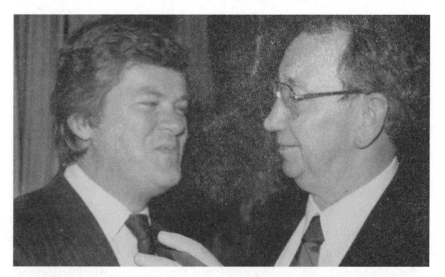

The Olympic bid was one of the few major issues in Alaska's recent history to
earn the support of both Anchorage newspapers. Gerry Grilly, publisher of the
Anchorage Daily News, and Bill Tobin, editor in chief of the *Anchorage Times*,
who were in mortal business combat with each other to see which of Anchorage's
two newspapers would survive, are shown here in the only existing picture of the
two together and smiling.

orage Times

GE WINS!

The next day the *Anchorage Daily News* banner headline blared, "Anchorage Gets Olympic bid" with the subhead "Delegation Wows Committee." The *Anchorage Times* front page shouted "ANCHORAGE WINS" with the subhead "We're America's Choice for the 1992 Winter Olympics." Their back-page banner headline was, "Mystrom delivers perfect pitch."

No one person made it happen but without some key Alaskans it would not have happened: among those critical to our success were the quietly strong Dave Baumeister; the confident-beyond-his-years Rick Nerland; the thoughtful, persistent Chris Swalling; the irrepressible Bob Penney; the creative Linda Chase; the popular and charismatic Chris Von Imhof; the deeply beloved Bill Tobin; the sometimes irritating, but very smart, aggressive, and hard-working Gerry Grilly; the influential senator Ted Stevens; and USOC member and Olympic swimmer Donna de Varona, who spoke strongly for Anchorage in the closed session preceding the vote.

We would later find out that we had won on the first round of voting, an almost impossible result with four qualified cities. In the Olympic world a secret vote is held with all candidates on the ballot. Typically, with four candidates, no candidate will get more than 50 percent so the lowest vote-getter is dropped and a second round of voting takes place. With three candidates usually no city will get more than 50 percent so once again the low vote getter is dropped and the final vote is taken with two cities. One city will then have a majority unless it is a tie. In that case the president of the USOC is allowed to vote and break the tie.

Our victory on the first round meant that we had received more than 50 percent of the votes on the first round—more than Salt Lake City, Lake Placid, and Reno-Tahoe combined.

Within a week I received a very gracious letter from Bill Martin, who coordinated the Reno-Tahoe bid. It said, in part:

> Dear Rick,
>
> ... We went to Indianapolis convinced we had the best package in terms of facilities, accommodations, and venues and, in all honesty, came home feeling the same way.
>
> But, in the words of one of our committee members, "It's like two guys asking the same girl to marry him and she picks the one she's in love with and not the one who can support her the best. "
>
> The USOC fell in love with Alaska and we wish you nothing but the best as you take your bid to the IOC. We'll vouch for your tenacity and spirit.
>
> Sincerely,
> Bill Martin, Coordinator
> Reno-Tahoe Organizing Committee

The USOC did fall in love with Alaska and Anchorage fell in love with the Bid Committee. The welcome home to Anchorage was held in a huge aircraft hangar and was a moment that no members of our committee will

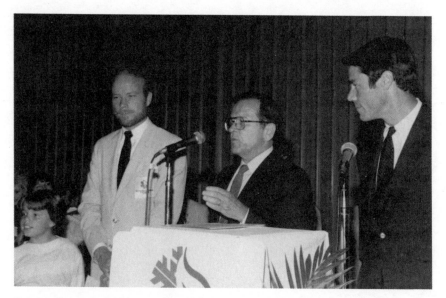

Senator Stevens speaking at the welcome-home event for the Anchorage Organizing Committee after the victory in Indianapolis. Anchorage mayor Tony Knowles is at right. Our daughter, Jenni, is at far left.

ever forget. But as in a marriage, the easy part is falling in love. The hard part is making it work. Now we had in front of us the challenge of persuading the International Olympic Committee around the world that Anchorage, Alaska could and should host the 1992 Olympic Winter Games.

During Anchorage's Olympic bids, it was crucial that I be sensitive to where my blood sugar was, especially at Olympic events and speeches around the world. That sensitivity to blood sugar levels and the relative urgency of corrective actions are important for any insulin-dependent diabetic.

Find a star, young man,
and follow it through the night.

T'will be a rare and mighty thing
you do if you keep it forever in sight.

You'll stumble and fall along the
way; your feet will be tired and sore.

Will you rise again and again
as so few have done before?

—"Follow a Star, Young Man," Susie Werner (1964)

Written just
after my getting
diabetes to
encourage me
to dream and
achieve despite
setbacks.

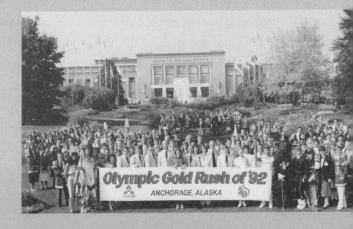

The nearly 200 Alaskans who traveled to Lausanne, Switzerland
in October 1986 to support Anchorage's bid for the 1992
Olympic Winter Games.

Chapter 11

Alaska's International Olympic Bids

America's Candidate for the Olympic Winter Games

After the Anchorage Organizing Committee's victory on June 15, 1985, we were officially America's candidate and the bid was restructured as America's bid. The level of support changed dramatically with the United States government putting its weight behind the bid. President Reagan became our honorary chairman. Secretary of State George Shultz was the top executive branch official for our bid and Alaska's senior senator Ted Stevens was the congressional leader for the bid.

I became the chairman of what was now America's bid. Dave Baumeister became the president and Rick Nerland became the secretary general (the international term for executive director).

We also had the strong support of Alaska senator Frank Murkowski, Alaska congressman Don Young, Alaska governor Bill Sheffield, and Anchorage mayor Tony Knowles. The support from our citizens was strong and the USOC was solidly behind us. Now we needed to earn the support of the majority of the International Olympic Committee voting members. Our goal was to persuade the IOC members of our enthusiasm for the Olympic Games, our commitment to Olympic ideals and our ability to organize and run the 1992 Olympic Winter Games. We were ready to go.

The International Olympic Committee

The governing body of the Olympics is the International Olympic Committee. At the time of Anchorage's Olympic bid the IOC had 92 voting members representing 60 countries. Each country that participates in the games has one representative and each country that has hosted at least one Olympics is entitled to one additional member. The United States, which had hosted at that time the Olympic Summer Games in St. Louis in 1904, in Los Angeles in 1932 and 1984, and in Atlanta in 1996, as well as the Winter Games in Lake Placid in 1932 and 1980, and in Squaw Valley in 1960, was entitled to two voting members. In North America, both Mexico and Canada had two votes as did more than a dozen countries in Europe and Asia. Australia also had two voting members.

The president of the International Olympic Committee was Juan Antonio Samaranch. President Samaranch, as he was addressed, had the second-longest reign as president of the IOC, second only to Pierre de Coubertin, the founder of the modern Olympics. Just prior to his election as president of the IOC, he was the Spanish ambassador to Russia. He was fluent in three languages: his native tongue of Spanish as well as English and French.

He was elected president of the IOC in 1980 just preceding the Olympics in Moscow and, by the time of our bid five years later, had already led the IOC to a much stronger financial position through the negotiation of television contracts primarily for the American television market and specifically with the ABC network.

Samaranch had a bit of a regal air about him that was sometimes criticized by the press but I found him to be very friendly and warm. Though he would be only one vote in the decision for the site of the Olympic Winter Games, his opinion was highly valued and carefully considered by other members. He was important to our strategy. Despite his friendliness and warmth toward me and despite the fact that he would periodically give me advice about our bid, I could never come to any definitive conclusions about his support or advocacy for Anchorage's bid.

Although the top staff of the United States Olympic Committee, under the leadership of General George Miller (ret.), were very supportive, I wasn't certain that Bob Helmick, the president of the committee, was privately supportive of our bid in the international competition. Publicly, Helmick was supportive and that was most important. I remember telling him early on that our Bid Committee was pretty new and a little naïve in this whole process and we would appreciate any advice he could give us. I recall his response as he was talking to a *New York Times* reporter later that day. As he recalled my comment he said, "The Anchorage committee is naïve all right. Naïve like a fox." Once again I felt we'd figure this competition out and could win.

Anchorage's Challenge

Anchorage had 15 months from the time we were selected as America's candidate for the 1992 Olympic Winter Games until the decision would be made at the annual meeting of the IOC in Lausanne, Switzerland on October 16, 1986.

Six cities were already in the competition by the time we were chosen: Falun, Sweden; Berchtesgaden, Germany; Cortina d'Ampezzo, Italy; Sophia, Bulgaria; Albertville, France; and Lillehammer, Norway. Anchorage was the seventh and last city to enter the competition. Not only did we have less time to get our message out to the 92 members of the International Olympic Committee in more than 60 countries, but we also had another big disadvantage. The United States had held the Winter Olympics in Lake Placid in 1980 just six years earlier and also held the 1984 Summer Olympics in Los Angeles just two years earlier. In addition to the recent games in the United States, Calgary, in western Canada and relatively close to Anchorage, would be the site of the 1988 Olympic Winter Games.

Three games in eight years would be in North America. And with the IOC's desire to spread the games around Europe, Asia, Australia, and North America, Anchorage was at an obvious disadvantage. We knew that. We also knew that Europe had 38 members compared to eight for North America (including Puerto Rico and Cuba). But we had been underdogs before and it made the challenge bigger and more fun.

Anchorage was ready. Enthusiasm was high and volunteers were flooding our office and our phones. Our fund-raising committee led by Penney,

Rasmuson, Brady, and Hickel had money flowing in daily. The media were supportive and our opponents were few and not very vocal.

Support also poured in from other Alaskan communities: the mayor of the Fairbanks North Star Borough, Bill Allen, was an enthusiastic and articulate supporter who helped rally Fairbanks to support the bid. The mayor of Juneau, the classy and intelligent Fran Ulmer, was a strong and up-front supporter and an influential force in Southeast Alaska. Polls were showing statewide support of over 80 percent which was even higher than the 75 percent support showing in Anchorage.

The Alaska Olympic Ambassadors Program
We divided the Olympic world into continents—Asia, Africa, North America, South America, Europe, and Australia (including New Zealand and the South Pacific), and assigned one or more executive committee members to each of those areas. As chairman, I had the broader responsibility of getting to know as many members as possible regardless of location.

After one of my trips to Asia which included meetings with seven IOC members in seven countries in nine days, I realized we needed to do something that would form deeper relations with the IOC members. In the shower, after I returned home, the solution came to me. We needed to create an ambassadors' corps of Alaskan volunteers. The mission of each ambassador would be to develop a friendship with their assigned IOC member and promote Anchorage to their IOC member.

Anchorage is such a diverse city I was sure that we could find 92 people or couples who had some connection with each of the countries. I also knew who could create and lead this program. That day I shared this concept with Dave Baumeister and Rick Nerland and told them that Duane and Carol Heyman were the ones who could make this program work.

Duane and Carol, as a team, had been volunteer leaders for a number of community groups including the Anchorage Symphony, the Alaska Light Opera, and the Anchorage Museum of History and Art. They were well connected and widely respected throughout Anchorage.

After we reviewed the concept with the executive committee of the board of directors, Rick approached the Heymans. Their answer was as firm and committed a "Yes" as I thought it would be. They took the concept and made it a reality. Within months the program was up and running with over 90 ambassadors who would, over the next five years, promote Anchorage's bid to IOC members at a personal level that would have been impossible for me or other members of the executive committee to achieve. Our ambassadors would spend thousands of dollars of their own money visiting their assigned member in his or her home country and then host their IOC members when they visited Anchorage. Many of the friendships made during the bids still exist today. It was an instrumental part of our bid and its success is directly attributable to the Heymans and the ambassadors themselves.

A few of the ambassadors who went way beyond any expectations were Eric and Vicki Sun-Chan who represented Anchorage to the People's Republic of China; Tom and Ruth Nighswander, who represented Anchorage to a number of different countries in Africa; and the bright and charming Sharon Gagnon, who represented Anchorage to both IOC members from France. José Vincent, who represented Anchorage to Brazil, and Ron and Karin Sheardown, who represented us to one of the Russian IOC members, were also very committed ambassadors for our bid.

The Olympics Are on the Ballot but I'm Not

Our Olympic Bid Committee wanted to have a citywide vote on hosting the Winter Olympics. We felt this was important for a number of reasons. A public vote would provide a reason and a forum to get information out. It would also give our supporters a chance to voice their support publicly and just as important, it would give our opponents a voice to air their opposition and our committee a chance to answer and rebut those concerns.

The proposition on whether or not the citizens of Anchorage wanted to host the Olympic Winter Games was voted on in Anchorage's regular municipal election October 1, 1985. It passed by a 2 to 1 margin.

Another issue in that election was the successor to my seat on the Anchorage Assembly. I had decided I would not run for a third term. During the campaign for the seat I was vacating, the *Anchorage Daily News* wrote an article headlined "Mystrom Is Role Model for Successor." The opening paragraph stated, "The four candidates running from the Spenard and Turnagain district are all busy trying to convince voters they are the next best thing to Rick Mystrom, who retires this year after six years on the job." I felt pretty good about that article until the following Tuesday night assembly meeting when Jane Angvik, the current assembly chairperson, my good friend and political opposite, said, "That article was a little much, Rick. You don't believe that bullshit, do you?"

Ya gotta love that woman. She says what she feels and she says it to you, not to others. Actually, that was one of her more R-rated comments. Many of her comments were more X-rated.

The two top candidates for my seat were both friends of mine, Bill Faulkner and Jim Kubitz. Bill won that night by 54 votes out of about 6,000 cast in that district. Jim won the race for the other seat in the district the next year. Both men were productive leaders on the assembly and both easily won reelection.

I was now officially out of political office. My advertising agency was continuing to grow under the leadership of Vice President Linda Boochever. Our kids were doing well in school and active in sports and I could devote more time to my new passion, Anchorage's Olympic bid.

Preparing for the IOC Decision

In the year leading up to the IOC decision scheduled for October 19, 1986 in Lausanne, Switzerland, our committee produced a spectacular promotional *bid* book and a 400-page comprehensive *technical* book that provided all the details of each venue and event. We produced dozens of brochures and began hosting national and international competitions in Nordic skiing, biathlon, alpine skiing, and hockey. We began working with the international governing bodies of each of the winter sports to understand what their needs were and how we could meet them. We also began communicating with all the national Olympic committees and began preparing presentations and exhibits for the Association of National Olympic Committees' annual meeting.

We organized scores of trips bringing IOC members to Anchorage to introduce them to our people, our city, and our layout for all the venues. The people of Anchorage opened up their hearts and homes and made wonderful and lasting impressions on the visiting members. One member, He Zhenlaiang, IOC member from China, after his visit to Anchorage made a comment to me that I have never forgotten. We were riding together on the way back to the airport after his visit to Anchorage. He turned to me and said, "Mr. Chairman, I've heard you speak at many meetings around the world but I've forgotten much of what you said. But when I saw your visual presentations, I remembered. Now that I've visited your city, I understand."

When you hear, you forget. When you see, you remember. But when you experience, you understand. That bit of wisdom is true and important and should be applied by anyone whose goal is to teach, inform, or persuade.

We began introducing Anchorage and Alaska to the Olympic world and world press. This effort resulted in many hundreds, maybe thousands, of articles, in newspapers and magazines and on television and radio stations around the world about Anchorage and Alaska. Certainly, Rick Nerland and his staff were the leaders that gave Anchorage such positive, worldwide recognition. The fascination with Alaska helped make their job a little easier but they knew that and used it well. In fact, our bid became known, not by the city and country as all other bids were, that is, Falun, Sweden; Albertville, France; Sophia, Bulgaria; Lillehammer, Norway; Berchtesgaden, Germany; and Cortina d'Ampezzo, Italy. We simply became known in the Olympic world as Anchorage, Alaska.

Under the day-to-day leadership of Dave Baumeister and Rick Nerland, the bid moved forward smoothly. The ambassadors program, under Duane and Carol Heyman, not only built relationships with IOC members but also gave us a huge amount of information about important IOC issues and other candidate city activities. We began to realize how important these relationships would be both for the successful operation of the games or for a second international bid if that were necessary.

We began hosting national and international competitions in cross-country skiing, alpine skiing, biathlon, figure skating, and hockey, all organized and superbly run by local volunteers. Every one of the events Anchorage hosted during the years leading up to our international bid exceeded all expectations. We got letter after letter from national and international sports governing bodies and from the US and international Olympic committees lauding the success of the events.

One particular event always brings a smile to my face. On March 2, 1986, the Anchorage Organizing Committee hosted an exhibition hockey game between the Norwegian and Yugoslav Olympic hockey teams. It was another success that exceeded all expectations.

After the game both Anchorage newspapers led their sports sections with big, positive stories. The *Anchorage Daily News* led with, "Norway, Yugoslav hockey teams a hit." The *Anchorage Times* proclaimed, "Olympic-Size Crowd Shows at Exhibition."

The *Times* story opened this way:

> With 4:42 left to play in Sunday's international hockey exhibition between Norway and Yugoslavia, a speeding puck deflected over the glass and headed for the seats. Of all the 6,014 fans at Sullivan Arena, it was Rick Mystrom, the driving force behind Anchorage's bid for the Winter Olympics, who made the circus catch. Protecting women and babes, he thrust the puck high and basked in the applause. Mystrom's gold-medal Midas touch lives. How else can the success of the Anchorage Organizing Committee's event be explained?

They ended their story by saying that the crowd roared for both teams … "but the real winner was the AOC."

Well, it was a clever opening and the "women and babes" part may have been hyperbole but the way that success could be explained was not by any Midas touch I had, but by the extraordinary efforts of Dave Baumeister and Tom Tierney, an AOC volunteer and hockey community leader. That event continued the streak of successful national and international competitions that were so important in showing the IOC Anchorage's ability to host top-quality international sporting events.

Although the *Times* called it a "circus catch" and the *Daily News* called it "a marvelous one-handed catch," Chris Grover, a high school student then and close friend of my son, Nick, saw it differently. When I bent down and handed the puck to a small girl sitting on a nearby aisle seat, Chris turned to Nick, sitting next to him, and said, "Nick, that puck has *governor* written all over it." It didn't. But the comment made me smile. Chris is now the head coach of the United States Cross-Country Ski Team.

Preparing the Presentation for the International Olympic Committee

With the bid itself in control and progressing well, I had been freed to chair the monthly board of directors and weekly executive committee meetings, work on continued statewide support, and visit IOC members personally. Now it was time to begin focusing on the presentation that I would make in Lausanne, Switzerland in October.

I spent many sunny afternoons walking the 12-block Park Strip, Anchorage's biggest downtown park, putting together the ideas in my head for the presentation. I'd make a complete lap, then return to the softball bleachers on the end nearest my office and write draft after draft of the presentation. The presentation was just one of many elements that would determine whether or not we would win. But it was the single element that would present its flaws or failure most obviously and most publicly. It had to be both logically persuasive and emotionally compelling. And the delivery had to be perfect.

From the press coverage following our victory in Indianapolis, I realized the impact that a strong presentation could have and I certainly didn't want to find out the damage a mediocre presentation could inflict on a bid. Over a period of a few weeks the presentation came together well. As in the US bid presentation, I planned on some rehearsal presentations before large Anchorage and statewide television audiences to build the Olympic spirit of Alaska and give us good feedback for the final presentation.

Anchorage's Human Olympic Rings

But for weeks, I struggled with the conclusion. What compelling vision could I end with that would demonstrate Anchorage's enthusiasm and support for the Olympics? Once again it was my morning shower that gave me the freshness to see the obvious. I visualized 5,000 volunteers on Anchorage's Park Strip in the shape of living Olympic rings with the date "1992" below the rings. Colored cards would be raised in the order of the Olympic logo: blue, yellow, black, green, and red and the year of the Games would appear below. Now I just had to find two leaders who could make it happen.

One of my choices was Don Dwiggins, an architect and community leader, who had led the University of California at Berkeley student card section when he was in college. The other was my wife, Mary, an excellent organizer, who had been looking for an Olympic project to take the lead in. They both enthusiastically agreed to take on the project when I asked.

I then called Roy Robinson, president of KFQD, the leader of Anchorage radio stations at that time. I asked Roy two questions. First, could he get all the stations to promote participation in the event? And second, how could we communicate simultaneously with all those people, spread over a full square block? The answer to the first question was "Yes" and the answer to the second question was just brilliant. He said he thought he could get every radio station in Anchorage to broadcast on the same frequency leading up to and during the event and he would provide Don and me with a mobile broadcast transmitter to direct the participants.

As the radio stations promoted the human Olympic rings, they all agreed to instruct volunteers to bring portable radios to the event. I would need to get the mayor and the fire chief to agree to let us use the city's biggest ladder truck. Don and I would be in the fire truck basket five or six stories up and could direct the timing of the cards. According to Roy, no matter what radio station anyone in Anchorage tuned into at that time they would hear Don or me saying "One, two, three blue; one, two, three yellow," and so forth.

I thought it could work. And it did. Don organized the outlines on the Park Strip and Mary organized the volunteer effort perfectly. Once again the AOC luck held. We had cold, rainy days leading up to the event. That morning, Mary and I worried about the turnout. But as if on call, the sun came out an hour before we started. The crowds swarmed into the area ready and, as we would find out, very excited.

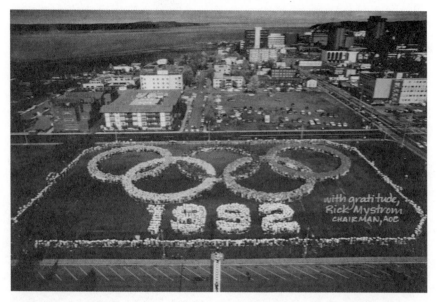

About 3,500 Anchorage citizens showed up at the Anchorage Park Strip on a Sunday afternoon, September 21, 1986, to show their support of our Olympic bid and become part of Anchorage's human Olympic rings. It was extraordinarily successful and became the conclusion of our presentation to the IOC.

Photo courtesy of Clark Mischler

Don and I were up in the basket of the ladder truck as we watched volunteers pass out 2-foot-square colored cards and direct all the card holders to their circles. From our vantage, we watched all the Olympic rings fill from left to right. Then the "1992" filled in. The balance of those who attended were directed around the border to complete the mural. Incredibly, the number of people who participated exactly filled the logo, the date, and the border.

As we prepared for the action, I gave some words of encouragement to the crowd. They were hyped and ready. I began, "One, two, three yellow," and at "Yellow" the yellow-card holders yelled out in a spontaneous cheer. From that point on it was electric. Every time I yelled out a color, those card holders tried their best to outyell the previous group. Photographers in planes and helicopters overhead recorded the visual dynamics and TV

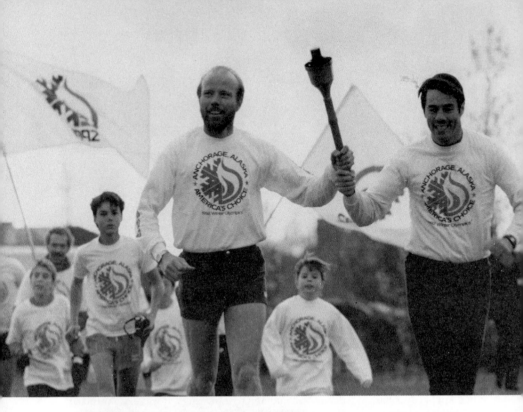

Top: The last leg of Alaska's Olympic torch relay as a final sendoff of the 200 Alaskans going to Lausanne, Switzerland to represent Alaska at the 91st session of the IOC. Mayor Tony Knowles and I carrying the torch together to light the awaiting bonfire.

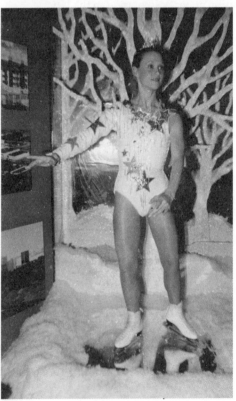

Left: One of the dozens of Olympic mannequins in Anchorage's very humanizing exhibition in Lausanne. The exhibit was designed and produced by Linda Chase's team and won the hearts of the Olympic family and the world press.

cameras on the ground captured the spirit and enthusiasm. And of course, every person listening to a radio in Anchorage had no choice but to hear what was happening.

The only glitch was my failure to check with Clark Mischler, our official event photographer, who was in one of the helicopters. After the fourth run-through, I felt the cheering had climaxed and it couldn't be louder or more enthusiastic. I thanked all the participants and dismissed them. As the living mural dissolved into a random crowd of fulfilled, buzzing people, I heard Clark yelling into my earphones, "I'm not done yet. I'm not done yet. Bring them back!" My reaction was it would be easier to put shaving lotion back into an aerosol can than it would be to get everyone to stop and recreate the mural. I didn't do it.

As it turned out, Clark had made all the great shots we needed to create a compelling conclusion to our presentation. Once again the people of Anchorage came through and so did our volunteer leaders.

Lausanne, Switzerland, October 15, 1986

We heard through our ambassadors program that a number of our international competitors knew we had brought 30 citizens to our presentation in Indianapolis when we won the American bid. They liked that idea and planned to bring similar-size groups of volunteers to Lausanne for their presentations. So we decided to bring 200. We had no problem lining up 200 volunteers, many of them our Olympic ambassadors, who wanted to take the trip to strengthen their relationship with their IOC members. Once again all the volunteers paid all their own expenses.

We had simple blue cotton parkas made for all the Alaskan attendees. Linda Chase and her crew put together another knockout exhibition highlighted by live mannequins representing all the Olympic winter sports. Bill Elander, the head of the Anchorage Convention and Visitors Bureau, paid for Anchorage's mascots, dancing moose and dancing bears, to attend and perform. But the highlight for the couple of hundred reporters there were the "Polar Bears." Not the white carnivores that roam the icepack north and west of Alaska, but the drink made famous in Alaska by the Anchorage Fur Rendezvous. It's a blended drink of vodka, kahlúa, and rich vanilla ice cream.

We soon realized the best place to promote Anchorage to the world press was in the Polar Bear line that sometimes stretched to 30 people with many repeat customers. While the Polar Bear line was a high-value target, our main targets were IOC members, so our executive committee and ambassadors were promoting our bid anywhere there was an IOC member.

The presentations for the winter cities were the third and final day of the IOC meeting. The summer cities would present the day before. This IOC session would be the last time the summer and winter cities would present at the same time. The IOC had approved a resolution that would, for the first time, alternate the Summer and Winter Games. The Summer Olympics would continue their four-year cycle and the Winter Olympics would be held in 1994 just two years after the 1992 Olympic Winter Games, and start a new four-year cycle of their own.

On the day of the presentation, all the Alaskans gathered on the main floor of the Palais de Beaulieu. As the eight-member official Anchorage delegation was called to go up the escalator into the main convention room holding the plenary session of the IOC, the 200 Alaskans who were there for support broke into a spontaneous rendition of the Alaska flag song led by Gloria Allen, our own opera diva. Now most Americans would say, "What? I don't even think my state has a flag song." But Alaska is different. We sing our flag song almost as often as we sing the national anthem. It concludes with the words, "… Alaska's flag to Alaskans dear, the simple flag of the last frontier." We may have been the only delegation that needed to wipe the tears away from our eyes as we entered the meeting room.

Anchorage mayor Tony Knowles did an excellent job leading off our presentation and then introduced me. My blood sugar was just under 200 mg/dl, almost 100 points higher than normal. In almost every other situation, I would have given myself two units of insulin to lower my blood sugar to my target of 100. For me each unit of insulin brings my blood sugar down 50 points. This is my adjustment factor. This, however, was not, a normal situation. I left my blood sugar there to remove any thought or concern about low blood sugar from my mind. If my blood sugar got too low, I would have to stop the presentation, drink the Seven-Up I had at the podium and wait for a minute or so to resume. That interruption would then become the defining moment of the presentation. I would not let that happen.

I opened the presentation:

> President Samaranch, ladies and gentlemen of the International Olympic Committee.
>
> The people of the city of Anchorage are proud to be here today to bid for the privilege of hosting the 1992 Olympic Winter Games.
>
> We recognize that the Olympic Winter Games will bring much to our city: a legacy of facilities for young athletes, a treasury of unforgettable memories, a wonderful feeling of community pride, and a deeper sense of international understanding.
>
> But we also know that Anchorage can bring much to the Olympic Winter Games:
>
> We bring to you today a city touched by the Olympic spirit, inspired by the Olympic challenge, and dedicated to protecting, enriching, and expanding the Olympic movement.
>
> Today you must not only decide which city has the best location, the best facilities, and the best venues to meet the qualifications of the Winter Games, but just as important, you must also decide which city has those special, unique qualities: the commitment, the enthusiasm, and the spirit that will make the Olympic movement stronger than ever before.
>
> Each of you in this room today have dedicated yourself to the Olympic movement. You are the custodians of its

past. You are the heart of its present. You are the architects of its future.

Soon you will choose the site for the 1992 Olympic winter games. A site that you believe will best carry forward Olympic ideals. A site that you believe will best protect and strengthen the Olympic movement.

We believe that site is Anchorage, Alaska.

I then went into the details of our site plan, our venues, our history of hosting events, and all the other details that demonstrated our ability to host the games. Then I finished this way.

Soon you will entrust one city with the honor of organizing the sixteenth Olympic Winter Games.

Soon you will entrust one city with the Olympic spirit. This spirit is priceless. It must be cherished.

The site you choose must be a place where the people of the world will put aside their differences and join together in a great celebration of peace and sport.

It must be a place whose people have the vision to dream the impossible and the ability to achieve it.

It must be a place so majestic it is inspiring, yet so beautiful it is humbling. There is, in the world, such a place.

This place is Alaska.

The lights went down and visions of Alaska in all its majesty filled the ballroom. The video ended with thousands of Alaskans on the Park Strip forming the human Olympic rings and the year, "1992."

When the lights came back up, I concluded with these words:

> At this very moment in Anchorage, Alaska, 250,000 people are waiting to hear your decision... waiting to find out if we have successfully shared with you our pride in our city, our enthusiasm for the Olympic Games, our commitment to Olympic ideals.
>
> Today you speak for the world. Your choice is difficult. But your responsibility is clear: to choose the city that can best protect, enrich, and expand the spirit, the enthusiasm, and the ideals of the Olympic movement.
>
> That city is Anchorage, Alaska. A young, vibrant, international city. A city whose people are filled with energy, excited by the challenge, united by the Olympic spirit, and prepared to welcome the world to the Olympic Winter Games in 1992.

I don't know how the other speeches were received but the applause was as loud and sustained as a group whose average age was in the mid 70s could muster.

Members of Anchorage's delegation who were in the room quickly left to pass on their excitement to the 200 or so who waited downstairs in the foyer. Our delegation wasn't alone in their reaction.

Harold Zimman from *Olympian Magazine,* who has attended every Olympiad since 1952, was quoted as saying, "I talked to about six IOC members and all of them said if the presentation determined the winner, then it would definitely be Anchorage."

James Worrall, IOC member from Canada, stated, "They were all very good this time [but] Anchorage was the best."

Tom Netter of the *Chicago Tribune* wrote, "Anchorage, one of seven cities seeking the Winter Games, produced perhaps the most spectacular final bid."

We had won the hearts of many of the people in Lausanne but had we won the votes of the IOC?

Bringing Honor to Anchorage

The decision for the host city for the 1992 Olympic Summer Games took place first. Over the past year two cities had emerged as the leaders, Paris, France and Barcelona, Spain. Paris had spent about $19 million on its bid and while I don't recall how much Barcelona spent it was probably in that ballpark.

The IOC's decision for the Summer Games was Barcelona. That decision was to have a significant impact on the Winter Games decision.

Two hours later all the winter candidate cities' contingents gathered in the auditorium on the main floor of the Palais de Beaulieu. President Samaranch entered the stage with other key members of the IOC executive committee.

Whenever I recall Samaranch walking toward the podium to announce the decision, it always brings to mind the story Bud Greenspan, an Olympic icon, wrote three weeks later for the *New York Times*. Bud was, at that time, the producer of the movie *Sixteen Days of Glory*, the definitive documentary about the 1984 Summer Games in Los Angeles. After that he produced documentaries of all Olympic Games until he died on Christmas Day 2010. In 1985 he had received the highest award given by the IOC, the Olympic Order. He was then and still is now considered the foremost writer, director, and producer of Olympic films.

Nobody has ever told the story of Anchorage's bid in Lausanne better than Bud Greenspan. The full-page *New York Times* opinion piece he wrote was titled "Bringing Honor to Anchorage." The story was introduced as follows by the *New York Times*:

> Bud Greenspan, author of this personal and warmly
> enthusiastic report on the dramatic impact made by
> Alaskans last month during the 91st meeting of the

International Olympic Committee in Lausanne,
Switzerland, is a power in both the entertainment and
sports world.

A movie producer and
director of great acclaim,
earlier this year he released
his documentary film
Sixteen Days of Glory,
which won acclaim for the
moving way in which it
captures the excitement
and drama of the 1984
Olympic Summer Games
in Los Angeles.

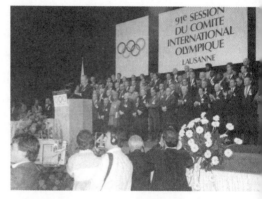

Here I'm making the presentation on
behalf of Anchorage and the United States
Olympic Committee to the International
Olympic Committee and the world press.

In Lausanne, Greenspan was able to see firsthand the
zest and vigor of the Anchorage pursuit of the Winter
Games. This report of his encounter with Alaskans in
Switzerland is scheduled later this month for national
publication and syndication.

Here are selected portions of the article titled "Bringing Honor to
Anchorage." The full text of his article appears in the appendix of this book.

One evening before you sit down to watch television
and have nothing better to do, pour yourself some
champagne or a stein of beer and raise your glass in a
toast to a marvelous group of Alaskans who did America
proud in Lausanne, Switzerland just three weeks ago.

There, this joyful contingent of more than 100 men and
women from Anchorage, most of whom paid their own
way, showed the high rollers and deal makers from six

other cities bidding for the 1992 Winter Olympic
Games what talent, pride, and courage is all about.

… The Anchorage people are America's present-day
pioneers. Some of them who came to Lausanne were
native-born Alaskans, but most of them originally came
from Chicago, Indianapolis, Salt Lake City, and
countless other places in the Lower 48 to make a life for
themselves in the new frontier.

… Brilliantly clothed in their white fur-trimmed blue
parkas and seemingly everywhere, the Anchorage
people were the most visible and enthusiastic group in
Lausanne. They knew their city was the "new kid on the
block" and they smiled the good smile as Gina
Lollobrigida was flown in to promote Cortina's bid and
watched respectfully as Prime Minister Jacques Chirac
of France joined triple gold medal winner Jean Claude
Killy in telling the world press why Albertville should
host the 1992 Winter Games.

There were no front-page superstars from Anchorage,
but their joy and vision brought more attention to their
presentation than any other city's bid.

… The beauty of the Anchorage people was their lovely
combination of professionalism and naiveté.
Overcoming insurmountable odds is part of the drill
when you become a pioneer. The main credo when you
enter the arena is that age-old axiom, "Some men see
things as they are and ask 'Why?' Others dream things
that never were and ask, 'Why not?'" So Alaskans asked,
"Why not?"

The people from Anchorage showed they were for real earlier this year in a preliminary IOC session in Seoul, South Korea, when a large group of Alaskans paid their own way in a dramatic show of support for the city's candidacy. They knocked the IOC members on their ears with their daring presentation which included the delightful antics of a tap-dancing moose.

However, besides the glamorous blue parkas and dancing moose, Anchorage had solid technical credentials to host the games. Its winter sports facilities are top drawer and second to none on this earth.

Furthermore, the Olympic Games are more than facilities, transportation, housing, athletes, and foreign spectators. The Olympic Games are people and not one of the candidates wanted the games more than Anchorage and all the Alaskan people.

What other bidding city could offer an untouched, beautiful wilderness just a half hour's drive from the Olympic sites with centuries-old glaciers creating a fantasy world with sight of magnificent Mount McKinley, the tallest mountain in North America?

When the Candidacy Committee of Anchorage led by its chairman, Rick Mystrom, the head of the largest advertising agency in Alaska, finished its presentation in Lausanne, its members were sure they had overcome the overwhelming obstacles that confronted them. Several IOC members promised their votes. Almost all of the Anchorage contingent ran to the telephones to send the word back home, certain they were going to pull the biggest upset in Olympic history.

For the next two days, they lobbied without really knowing how to lobby—just sheer joyful exuberance that was contagious. They did not know or believe that those same IOC members who promised votes were speaking from the emotion of the moment and would later reflect that their "real world" commitments were elsewhere.

… Two nights before the voting, the Alaskans held a dinner to honor their candidacy committee and supporters. Before the dinner there was a cocktail party that was more like a victory rally before a Notre Dame football game.

Each speaker was cheered to the rafters and the momentum of their fervor was intoxicating, and for a moment even I began to think that perhaps there might be justice in the world and God would smile down on this happy band of Alaskans.

So I asked Rick Mystrom to invite his contingent to a screening of *Sixteen Days of Glory*, our film on the 1984 Los Angeles Olympic Games that was scheduled to be shown the next morning to the world press just a few hours before the announcement of the winning Olympic cities.

I thought this would be my contribution to their effort… to have two hours watching the grandeur and glory of the greatest of athletic events and to perhaps reflect, win or lose, on the nobility of what they had done and what they must continue to do.

When the film was over, many (with tears in their eyes) came over to me laughing and crying, and for a brief moment were sober in their thoughts. My last words to them were those that sent the ancient Greeks into the Olympic arena so many years ago: "Ask not alone for victory, ask for courage, for if you endure, you bring honor to yourself, even more you bring honor to us all."

At that point I believe many of them for the first time realized that perhaps their time was not 1992 but 1994.

The Decision

I studied Samaranch as he walked up to the podium to make the announcement. His quiet confidence and upright posture gave him a look of strength despite his small stature. Samaranch said nothing for at least 10 seconds. The room, with members of all seven competing cities, sitting in their own groups, was completely silent. Samaranch made no introductory comments. He picked up a sealed envelope that had been placed on the podium, tore it open, looked up and announced: "Albertville."

> After the voting was over, one reporter came over to Rick Mystrom and asked what he and his Alaskans were going to do. Speaking for all of them, he replied, "We'll get home on Sunday, take Monday off, and on Tuesday start working for 1994."

> So one night when you've got nothing better to do, raise your glass in a toast to that happy band of Americans from Anchorage, those pioneers who entered the arena, dreamed a dream and fought the good fight. For one week in Lausanne they showed the world what American pioneers were like those many years ago. And because of it they brought honor to us all.

> —*Bud Greenspan*

Albertville, France had won. The conventional wisdom was that because Paris had not won the Summer Olympics, the IOC members had appeased the French by selecting Albertville as the site of the Winter Olympics. Though I have no firsthand information on that rumor, the logic was believable.

The dynamics of any vote with multiple candidates can influence an outcome almost as much as the merit of the candidates. According to Bud Greenspan and others, we were hindered by the fact that Montreal and Los Angeles were summer hosts in 1976 and 1984 and Lake Placid and Calgary were winter hosts in 1980 and 1988. Had we won, North America would have then received the Olympic bid five times within a 16-year period.

The most enduring and perhaps, by that measure, the most deserving of the competing cities for the 1992 Winter Games was Falun, Sweden. Falun had bid twice before and in the past a number of cities had been selected on their third bid. Their candidacy was headed by Lars Eggertz. Mary and I had become friends with Lars and his wife Anna Marie, after we hosted their son Daniel when he visited Alaska. Lars had committed 10 years of his life to bringing the Olympics to Falun and the loss that night was very hard on him and the whole Swedish delegation.

Another IOC vote that took place in Lausanne at that meeting was the election of Anita De Frantz as the second member of the IOC from the United States. Anita was an Olympic medalist in rowing and had been awarded the IOC's Bronze Medal of the Olympic Order for her stand against President Carter's US boycott of the 1980 Summer Olympics in Moscow—a boycott initiated, ironically, because of the Russian occupation of Afghanistan. At 31 she was also the youngest member ever voted in as an IOC member. She was the first American woman on the IOC and in 1997 became the first female vice president of IOC executive committee.

Anita had already advised us and helped us with our bid for the 1992 games and would, in a very short period of time, become a highly regarded IOC member and a valuable advocate for Anchorage in our upcoming bid for the 1994 Winter Games.

Now for the first time in Olympic history a candidate to host the next Olympic Winter Games would be chosen in two years instead of four.

Our Bid for the 1994 Olympic Winter Games

Our delegation returned to Anchorage on October 19, 1986 to a huge and enthusiastic crowd in a hangar at Anchorage International Airport chanting "Ninety-four, ninety-four, ninety-four!" It was an unforgettable and a very inspiring moment for all the returning Alaskans. I know I was certainly inspired and ready to go to work for the next bid.

The first task was to get the USOC to reelect Anchorage as America's candidate. The USOC meeting was scheduled for November 22 and 23 in Reno/Sparks Nevada. Five other American cities had expressed an interest in becoming America's candidate: Denver, Portland, Lake Placid, Reno-Tahoe, and Salt Lake City, but Anchorage was selected unanimously or very nearly so, as I recall.

Now we were ready to begin the process of preparing for the 1994 bid, which would take place in Seoul, South Korea in September 1988 at the Summer Olympic Games.

We put together a financial plan for the new bid. We had spent $2.5 million, the least of the seven cities competing for 1992. The other cities spent the following amounts (converted to American dollars) on their bids:

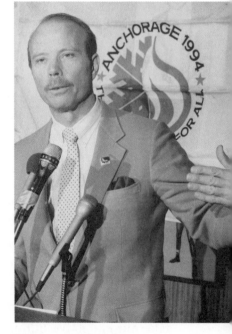

Falun, Sweden .... $12 million

Albertville, France .... $7 million

Berchtesgaden,
West Germany .... $7 million

Lillehammer, Norway ...... $5 million

Cortina d'Ampezzo, Italy ... $5 million

Sophia, Bulgaria .... $3 million

Anchorage, Alaska .... $2.5 million

Making one of my first Olympic speeches after losing in Lausanne and then winning the USOC's support to be America's candidate for the 1994 Olympic Winter Games.

To the best of my knowledge we were the only city financing its bid entirely with private money. Most of the money spent on the other cities' bids came from national or provincial governments.

We thought we could put together a successful bid for the 1994 Winter Olympics for about the same amount as we did for 1992 even though we were the most parsimonious of the cities. That decision was a result of two factors: (1) We had much of the work already done, and (2) Alaska was in the midst of a great economic collapse.

The price of oil, the driver of Alaska's economy, had collapsed in 1986 from $30 a barrel to $9 a barrel. Anchorage lost 13 percent of its population and 25 percent of its assessed valuation. Thirteen banks had failed or were failing and thousands of people had lost their homes.

In 1985, one of my companies, American Multiplex, owned nine commercial buildings (eight apartment buildings and one downtown office building) in Anchorage. To follow the apartment market, I counted classified ads in both newspapers every Sunday. (This was before Craig's List and other Internet options). That year I had seen a dramatic increase in apartments for rent in the classified sections. Based on that, I decided to sell a major part of my real estate holdings. Because the rental market was coming off a strong year, the apartments and the downtown office building sold quickly. I sold five of my buildings and kept four, so our family was okay. That wasn't the case, however, with all our key volunteers. Even as they were working on our bid, some were losing their homes.

Every day seemed to bring more and more bad economic news. Businesses were closing, banks failing, savings and loans going under, and people were moving out of Alaska to find work. As a result, the Olympic bid took on an additional identity. The Olympic bid was a ray of economic hope. Something good to talk about and something to take our collective minds off the financial problems that so many Alaskans were feeling. It was the only good dream out there amid our economic nightmare.

Many Alaskans, through letters to the editors of both newspapers and personal notes to committee members, spoke of how important the Olympic bid was during this time of financial hardship in our state. Of all the letters one particular letter provided inspiration and motivation to me throughout our bids:

2/24/88

Rick:

You are incredible—saw you at the Chamber this week. You are a constant inspiration to so many in this city with your selfless devotion to public service and to making Anchorage a better place to live today. While so many of us are discouraged by the financial destruction around us, you see positives. In fact you create the positives. I noticed the power of your speaking. You put yourself solidly on the line. You commit. There was no "If we are successful in bringing the Olympics here." It was "when" and "after." You are an irresistible force which nothing can move from his objective. Many of us will support you in anything you want to do to contribute.

Love from all of us.

This was a note I kept visible during some of the long, tough, and periodically disheartening times. It made the tough times easier and the good times more joyous. Unfortunately, I don't recall who wrote the note nor do I recall who "Love from all of us" refers to. But to whoever wrote it, thank you for those kind and inspirational words.

Our committee knew that in this debilitating economic environment we couldn't expect to raise much more than we had raised before. We decided on a budget of $3 million and got to work.

In addition to the work of our fund-raising committee, State Senator Tim Kelly, who sadly died too young, drafted a bill that allowed every Alaskan who applied for a Permanent Fund Dividend (an annual dividend paid to Alaskans based on earnings from a fund created from royalties paid to the state for oil extraction) to check off a donation of $10 to be subtracted from that person's dividend. That bill passed both houses of our legislature and resulted in well over 100,000 Alaskan citizens donating to our bids. Although Senator Kelly made that happen, the idea originated with Bob Penney. At the start of our bid Bob had told me he'd have boatloads of ideas. "Nine out of ten," he said, "will probably be bad, but if you can pick out the great ones we'll be successful." This was one of the great ones.

We had the organization in place with no major changes from the previous bid. We tuned and upgraded some of our venue proposals. We continued the highly successful ambassadors program. We prepared new videos and brochures. We began preparing new exhibits for the international meeting leading up to the decision. We hosted national and international governing bodies for all the winter sports. We continued planning and hosting national and international competitions.

Alaska's lone congressman, Don Young, led our congressional delegation's effort to get the State Department more active in our bid. The State Department agreed to provide an official presence at meetings between the Anchorage Organizing Committee and the IOC. They also agreed to maintain regular embassy contact with IOC and national Olympic committee members of countries participating in the Olympics. Governor Sheffield strongly supported our bid and his successor, Governor Steve Cowper, continued that support. Senator Frank Murkowski stepped up to the plate promoting our bid internationally and throughout the state of Alaska. And Anchorage's new mayor, Tom Fink, played a key role as well.

A Major Controversy for Our Bid Committee

Any major project with the potential to change the image and reality of a city is bound to have some controversy. For the Olympic bid the controversy focused around the traditional responsibility of the host city to cover a financial loss, if any, incurred in the hosting of the Olympics.

This requirement was in the Olympic Charter, which we gave to the press early on in the bid. However, in 1978 Los Angeles was the only city bidding for the Summer Olympics and a city charter amendment prohibited

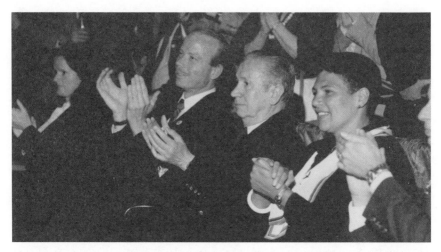

Juan Antonio Samaranch, president of the International Olympic Committee, *center;* Anita De Frantz, *right,* newly elected member of the IOC from the United States; and me during their visit to Anchorage to review our bid sites.

the use of city funds to organize the games. Because of that, Los Angeles could not guarantee the games with public funds. The International Olympic Committee waived the requirement in its charter and allowed the Los Angeles Olympics to hold the 1984 games with no public guarantee. That was the most recent position by the IOC as we began our bid in 1985.

The LA model was our model also, only on a smaller scale, since the Winter Olympics are quite a bit smaller than the Summer Olympics. LA operated their games without public guarantees and finished with a surplus. We could too. Television revenues were a huge part of their financial success. Their Pacific time zone was excellent for the American television networks. We had a similar advantage. But our Alaska Time zone was even one hour better than theirs for televising Olympic events throughout America. The importance of this was confirmed when the 1988 Winter Games in Calgary, which has a time zone almost as favorable as ours, received $309 million for television rights compared to $300 million that same year for the 1988 Summer Olympics in Seoul, which did not have a favorable time zone—this despite the fact that the Summer Games are about 10 times larger than the Winter Games. We felt certain we could organize a successful, privately funded event.

As noted earlier, in 1985, very early in our international bid for the 1992 Winter Olympics, Anchorage had an advisory vote to determine whether or not the citizens supported hosting the games. In that vote, Anchorage residents voted 2 to 1 in favor of going forward with the bid. About three years later during our bid for the 1994 Winter Olympics the financial guarantee became a major issue. The IOC by that time had issued a new contract assuring that privately funded games as in LA in 1984 would not be allowed to happen again. The issue was amplified by the fact that at an AOC Board meeting I said that the guarantee issue was not discussed by our committee until *after* the first vote in 1985.

About four days after that board meeting, I got a call from Rick Nerland. He asked me to stop by the AOC office on my way home from work. When I got there all his staff was gone and we sat down in the reception area. He showed me a yellow tablet on which he, as the executive director, had listed the agenda for discussion at an executive committee meeting about three years earlier. One of the subjects was "Guarantee Issue." It was dated four days *before* the first election. I was wrong. We had discussed it just before the first election.

I didn't know what that discussion, prior to the vote, entailed. But now I did know that we had discussed it and I had said we hadn't. It never occurred to either Rick or me that we just not say anything about that discovery. The first thing I said to Rick was, "I need to call the newspaper right away and tell them I was wrong."

That night after dinner, I called Howard Weaver, the managing editor of the *Anchorage Daily News*, at his home. I told him what Rick Nerland had discovered and my statement that we had not discussed the issue prior to the first vote was incorrect. I remember Howard's exact words: "This must be a hard call for you to make, Rick. Not many would have done it." He then said that he would have a reporter call me in the morning to discuss the issue.

I discussed the issue with a reporter the following morning. When the story came out the headline was something like "AOC Chief Admits He Knew of Guarantee before Vote." It wasn't until the last line in the story that it said, "When Mystrom realized his error, he immediately called the newspaper."

That story raised a month-long furor. We quickly called a special AOC board meeting and decided to have another vote on the willingness of the citizens of Anchorage to support the bid *with* a financial guarantee. That vote, on August 23, 1988 passed with the same 2 to 1 margin as the first vote and served to reinforce Anchorage's commitment to the Olympics.

The Proximity of the Calgary Games—an Advantage and Not

We were able to take advantage of the Winter Olympics in Calgary in February 1988. The Nordstrom Corporation rented the Anchorage Organizing Committee their corporate jet, which gave us a great opportunity to shuttle IOC members attending the Calgary games to Alaska and back every two days. Once we got the IOC members to Alaska, the Ambassadors once again played a key role in representing our city to the IOC. I traveled to Calgary multiple times during those games but saw only one event plus the parade. While in Calgary, I heard from a number of IOC members that Jean Claude Killy, who had been instrumental in Albertville's win, had spoken early and often to European IOC members about Anchorage being the best choice for the 1994 games.

As Mary and I and some other members of our delegation were watching the parade, I noticed that leading the parade was a lively, somewhat casual group of 80-year-olds. I turned to Dick Angell, a member of our delegation, and said, "Dick, who are those guys?" He smiled and said, "They're the surviving members of Calgary's original Bid Committee." Mary and I both laughed—but for just a moment. I think we both visualized a similar scene in Anchorage.

While the Calgary games gave us an opportunity to show Anchorage to a number of IOC members, the proximity did cause some concern from some members as the vote approached.

Though I've been unable to confirm it, I did hear from more than one Calgary volunteer that a poll was taken following the Olympic Games. The results as relayed to me were as follows: 92 percent said hosting the Olympics was great for Calgary; 6 percent said it was bad for Calgary; and 2 percent said "What Olympics?"

The Decision for the 1994 Winter Olympics

We were more experienced, well prepared, and quietly confident going into the final days before the decision for the 1994 Winter Olympics. The night before the decision, our staff had set up a series of 15-minute meetings for me with IOC members in the Shilla Hotel in Seoul, where Mary and I as well as the IOC members were staying. Between meetings I was in our room rehearsing the presentation I would make before the IOC the next day. People were in and out of our room in a flurry of frenetic activity. My voice was getting hoarse. Mary pulled me aside and asked, "How are you doing? How's your blood sugar? Are you okay?" I remember telling her I had just checked my blood sugar and it was fine. Then I said something that I'll always remember. I said, "This is living, Mary. I feel really alive."

It was a self-revealing comment that I've reflected on over the years. I realize how much I thrive on pressure and how many times I've been in high-pressure situations and felt energized by the challenges of them. I wouldn't want to be in those situations every day but I welcome them when they arrive.

Only four cities were competing this time: Ostersund, Sweden; Sophia, Bulgaria; Anchorage, Alaska; and Lillehammer, Norway.

Once again I made the presentation on behalf of Alaska and the United States. On stage with me and having roles in the presentation were Undersecretary of State Edward Derwinsky, Senator Frank Murkowski, and Anchorage mayor Tom Fink.

This time I started with a message of the friendship that had developed among the four competing cities.

> President Samaranch, ladies and gentlemen of the
> International Olympic Committee.
>
> ... Tomorrow you have the difficult task of choosing
> one city from among the four candidate cities. And we
> hope the city you choose will be Anchorage. But this
> week I have worn on my lapel the pins of all four cities
> because we have all become friends. We have all
> become better cities.

The people of Anchorage thank you for all your work
to help create world peace and understanding
through sport.

... And now I would like to begin our presentation
with a message from a great supporter of the Olympic
movement, President Ronald Reagan.

After President Reagan's videotaped message concluded, I continued
with our message about the successful competitions we had hosted during
the past two years. I showed our equidistance by air from Asia, Europe,
and the population centers of North America. I talked about our average
daylight in late February, more than the average daylight of all previous
Winter Olympic cities, and our February temperature—an average high
of 17.7 degrees Fahrenheit, ideal for winter competitions.

I presented our package of competition sites: A ski area considered
excellent for competition and with a major new luxury hotel planned (which
has since been built). I showed our Nordic ski facility, Kincaid Park, considered the best cross-country competition site in the United States, and
our hockey sites. Alaska at that time had three of the five Olympic-size
hockey rinks in America (NHL rinks are smaller than Olympic rinks).

I also talked about the venues that we would build, a very important
consideration to the IOC because they don't necessarily want to have the
Olympics in a city that has all the facilities in place. They favor a city that
has to build more venues and will therefore promote the opportunity for
growth of winter sports.

The presentation then went into a spectacular video featuring the
majesty of Alaska beautifully produced by David Haynes, Kathy Dunn,
and Cheryl Tatum.

I concluded with a slight variation of my 1992 conclusion:

... Your choice is difficult but your challenge is clear: to
choose the city that will best protect, enrich, and expand
the Olympic movement.

We believe that city is Anchorage, Alaska. A young,
vibrant, international city. With an ideal location. In a
beautiful setting. A city whose people are filled with
energy, excited by the challenge, united by the Olympic
spirit, and committed to welcoming the world to a great
Olympic Winter Games in 1994.

When I finished the presentation, the IOC posed only one question. That question, regarding Anchorage's August 23 vote, was answered by Mayor Fink. He told the IOC that the 2 to 1 margin was far wider than his victory margin in the mayoral election. The *Anchorage Times* quoted Flip Todd, a member of the Anchorage contingent as saying, "That explanation produced a big laugh from the IOC members. The mayor handled that beautifully."

On the first round of voting the totals were as follows: Lillehammer had 25 votes, Anchorage had 23, Ostersund 19, and Sophia 17. Sophia as the low vote-getter was dropped and a second round of voting took place. The question was what would happen with Sophia's votes. It was widely assumed that most of Sophia's votes were from Soviet bloc countries and with the Cold War still in play, none of their votes would go to the US candidate and not many would go to Norway, a western-aligned nation and a member of NATO. That's exactly what happened. None of the votes went to Anchorage and most went to Sweden, a more neutral nation than Norway or the United States.

In that second round of voting Sweden gained 14 of Bulgaria's votes to move ahead with 33 votes. Norway gained only five votes and moved into second with 30 votes. Anchorage, as the US candidate, had no prayer of getting any of the Soviet bloc votes and actually dropped one vote to 22. That meant Anchorage was out. In the third and final round, 15 of our votes went to Norway, 6 went to Sweden and one of our supporters apparently didn't vote for either one.

Lillehammer had beaten Sweden by six votes and Anchorage had finished third. We had lost for the second time. This time we were much closer: 23 votes in the first round compared to seven votes two years earlier but that didn't ease the disappointment. Many of our volunteers by that time had committed four years to the effort to bring the Olympics to Anchorage and I honestly don't recall a single one saying, "That's it for me. I'm done." The spirit and the willingness of our volunteers, and of a large majority of all Alaskans, to go for the Olympic Winter Games one more time was a great source of inspiration for all those who had given so much for so long in our attempts.

We were also inspired by the reaction of many of the IOC members who came up to me and others on our Bid Committee to say, "Next time is Anchorage's turn." One influential European member, referring to Europe, told me, "Now we [Europe] will have two games in a row; 1998 will go to Anchorage for sure." And from an Asian member, "You have made so many friends on the IOC, surely 1998 will go to Anchorage." All together we had counted more than 24 such comments.

Not only were the comments from the IOC encouraging but each of our competitors said Anchorage would be the next winner. Some, like the Swedes, said it with an echo of sadness because they realized they would not see the games for at least 30 years.

None of us on the executive committee were naïve enough to believe that those comments meant firm commitments. But it was an encouraging starting point and the logic was believable. Europe had almost half the votes and certainly those voters' provincial interests were at play, but the desire to maximize revenue and to spread the Olympic movement to all parts of the world is also a key element of most decisions.

An Anchorage victory would help achieve both those ends—spreading the Games around and maximizing revenue. If Anchorage were to win the 1998 bid, it would be the first time in 14 years that any Olympic Games would be held in America. And by now the IOC knew that Anchorage would provide the best opportunity for live television coverage across the United States. The importance of that factor was illustrated by the size of the TV contracts for the 1988 Calgary Winter Olympics. The Canadian TV rights brought $153 million to the Olympic movement and the American TV rights brought $309 million to Olympic coffers. All the other TV rights worldwide combined brought in less than $20 million.

Because Alaska's time zone is two hours more advantageous than even Calgary's good time zone, Anchorage would bring more television revenue to the Olympic movement than any other winter city ever. A 4 p.m. Olympic event in Anchorage is prime time across America. The American TV networks referred to it as "Anchorage's marvelous time zone," and they were very supportive of us because of it.

Both Bob Helmick and Anita De Frantz, the IOC's two American members said they were encouraged by Anchorage's showing in Seoul. "Anchorage didn't lose," Helmick said, as the Lillehammer group chanted the name of their city and waved a Norwegian flag. "Anchorage is a big winner. By being a close second in the first round, the vote made before any possible political deals take effect, Anchorage showed its strength." He followed that by saying, "I think the first-round vote is what really indicates the true strength of Anchorage's bid. What it indicates, indeed, is that Anchorage has the capability of winning the games."

Anita DeFrantz, now America's senior member of the IOC and a highly respected leader in the Olympic movement, said the AOC shouldn't be disappointed. "They did extremely well," she said. "They have the respect. They have the trust and they have the confidence of the IOC."

On a lighter note, Senator Frank Murkowski said in a letter to Mary and me about a week later:

Dear Rick and Mary,

I was extremely proud of the way our team in Seoul went about its task. Although pitted against heads of state and heads of government, the Anchorage group carried out a campaign that lacked nothing in its professionalism. If Anchorage were a country, it would have one of the world's most effective diplomatic corps. Your leadership was reflected in every aspect of the operation.

Sincerely,
Frank H. Murkowski
United States Senator

Not only did we have strong support from the IOC for our 1998 bid but we had continuing support from our citizens. Here is just one letter of the hundreds we received from supportive Alaskans:

> Dear Mr. Mystrom,
>
> Although you do not know me personally, I am one of the many Alaskans you and the Anchorage Organizing Committee represent when presenting Anchorage to the world. This letter is handwritten because I want you to know how sincere I am when I say what a phenomenal job you and the AOC did on presenting our city and state.
>
> Although we did not win the '94 bid for the Olympics this time, I speak for a lot of people when I ask you and the other members of AOC to please keep trying. The next time we're sure to win.
>
> I did watch the presentation you gave on Alaska and Anchorage to the IOC in Seoul, South Korea and I mean it when I say I have never felt more proud of Anchorage, Alaska, her people and the people who, like yourself, represented us in such a true-to-life way. It makes me feel good that I've chosen Alaska for my home.
>
> God bless you, Mr. Mystrom and the other members of the AOC. It's nice to know that there are other Alaskans out there who love and believe in Alaska as much as I do and who recognize the potential our city has.
>
> I realize you and the AOC have put a lot of time, effort, and money into the 1994 bid and it was well worth it. I ask you now to please consider bidding for the 1998 Olympics. We're sure to win next time.

Not that it means a lot but for whatever it's worth you have my support for the 1998 Olympics. Nothing can stop us now.

Sincerely,
Casey Ogren
Anchorage, Alaska

We had strong support at home and with the International Olympic Committee. As had been the case with Calgary, which had won the games on its third try, it was becoming more and more apparent that 1998 was going to be Anchorage's year to host the Olympic Winter Games. We had only one more hurdle to clear. We needed the USOC to renominate Anchorage as America's candidate for 1998.

The USOC meeting and decision was scheduled for June 3 and 4, 1989 in Des Moines, Iowa.

A Change in Leadership of the AOC

Before we began preparation for that meeting, I spent a lot of time reflecting on whether I could keep up my energy for another four years as chairman of our Bid Committee. For nearly five years I had been chairman of the committee for our three bids to date: The first for the USOC nomination, the second for the 1992 games and the third for the 1994 games. To continue as chairman would mean another bid to the USOC and then a final bid to the IOC for the 1998 games.

I was also the president and CEO of Mystrom Advertising and between the two jobs—one paid and one volunteer—I was working 50 to 60 hours a week with very little time off. I wasn't sure I could keep that same level of commitment as AOC chairman for the next four and a half years.

I talked with Dave Baumeister, the AOC president. Dave felt that the press of his corporate business wouldn't allow him to increase his time commitments to the bid but we agreed that Chris Swalling would be a good choice for chairman.

We made the recommendation to the nominating committee. They concurred and at our board of directors meeting on December 14, 1988, Chris was elected chairman. I agreed to stay on as a member of the Executive Committee, act as chairman of the International Relations Committee, and make the presentation to the USOC in June 1989. That night the committee held a wonderful event to thank Mary and me for our commitment to our bid over the past five years. Over the next few weeks I received many kind, supportive, and encouraging letters from members of the International Olympic Committee as well as from citizens of Alaska.

My journey as chairman of Anchorage and America's bids hadn't ended the way I hoped and envisioned but what a ride it had been—being immersed in the national and international Olympic movements, meeting hundreds of bright, interesting, and dedicated people; representing America and Alaska around the world, experiencing the thrill of victory and the disappointment of defeat. But through it all the most inspiring part was the generous, enthusiastic, and enduring support of my fellow Alaskans and especially the citizens of Anchorage who gave so much for so long. With no reward other than renewed pride in their city and the knowledge that they stepped into the arena, dreamed a good dream, and fought a good fight. They endured and because of it they brought honor to us all.

I experienced personally the truth in Teddy Roosevelt's memorable quote: "Far better to dare mighty things, to win glorious triumphs, even though checkered by failure, than to take rank with those poor spirits who neither enjoy much nor suffer much, because they live in the gray twilight that knows neither victory nor defeat."

In January 1989 we began preparing for the United States Olympic Committee's June meeting to select America's candidate for the 1998 Olympic Winter Games. Since I was then chairman of the International Relations Committee, my role was continuing our relationships with the IOC members. I had a more limited role in working with USOC members and the various national governing bodies of Winter Sports.

The AOC, under Chris's leadership and with the support and leadership of Dave Baumeister and Rick Nerland, dedicated itself to promoting our bid to the USOC and building support for our candidacy. Bud Greenspan once again came to Anchorage's aid by producing an inspirational film that told the story of three different Winter Olympic athletes who didn't medal on their first two tries but won the gold on their third try.

In making our presentation to the USOC on behalf of Anchorage, I stressed the fact that over one third of the IOC members had, by that time, told us, "This is Anchorage's time." "Now is Anchorage's moment." They told us we had worked four years against great odds and we had earned the right to host the games. They told us how much they appreciated the enthusiasm and spirit we had brought to the Olympic movement. They told us that our people had won the hearts of the IOC—and many had told us that in 1998, Anchorage would host the Olympic Winter Games.

I also talked about the facilities we had and the facilities we would build, the successful competitions we had held, and our complete venue plan for the games. I stressed the point that the only other international competitor entered so far was Nagano, Japan and they would have a two-year head start against any American city other than Anchorage.

After all four American cities, Denver, Reno-Tahoe, Salt Lake City, and Anchorage made their presentations, we had only a short wait.

In less than two hours, the decision was announced: Salt Lake City had won. While I don't know the exact total, the *New York Times* reported it was very close and required a second vote to decide between Salt Lake City and Anchorage.

After the vote, I told the press that I thought the 1998 games would go to Nagano. I was right about that.

Nagano won for the 1998 Winter Games and four years later, Salt Lake City won for the 2002 games. I also told the press that though it was close, the Salt Lake City Organizing Committee had beaten us "fair and square." I was wrong about that.

More than 10 years later we found out how Salt Lake City had beaten us.

The Bribery Scandal That Shook
the Olympic Movement Worldwide

On December 10, 1998, highly respected and longtime Swiss IOC member Marc Hodler, who was head of the committee overseeing the organization of the 2002 Games, revealed that several IOC members had taken bribes from the Salt Lake City Organizing Committee. Both the International Olympic Committee and the United States Olympic Committee began investigations. Soon after that the U.S. Department of Justice began an investigation.

The Salt Lake City corruption investigation resulted in at least five members of the IOC being expelled, four other IOC members resigning, and 10 other IOC members being sanctioned.

In December 1998, the United States Olympic Committee appointed a special commission to investigate alleged improprieties related to the selection of Salt Lake City over Anchorage to become America's candidate for the 2002 Winter Olympics.

Federal prosecutors filed 15 federal felony charges against the leaders of the Salt Lake City Bid Committee, Tom Welch and Dave Johnson. Testimony in the trial of Welch and Johnson revealed information about their competition against Anchorage for the United States' candidacy. The testimony revealed that they had paid a key USOC member, Alfredo LaMont, to gather and deliver to them information he had access to, as a USOC member, about Anchorage's bid. Also according to testimony in that trial, as reported by the *Deseret News* (a major Salt Lake City newspaper) Welch and Johnson paid LaMont to use his USOC influence to gain votes for Salt Lake City in their competition against Anchorage. All this was happening leading up to our razor-thin loss to Salt Lake City.

According to the *Deseret News*, Nov. 20, 2003,

> LaMont acknowledged he failed to pay $175,000 in taxes in
> 2001, a year after he pleaded guilty to two tax felonies,
> including one involving earnings from the Salt Lake
> bid.… Initially, LaMont provided information he collected,
> as a USOC employee, about Anchorage, Alaska, and other
> U.S. cities competing against Salt Lake City. Later, he also
> tapped his international contacts for information to boost
> Salt Lake's campaign. The arrangement between LaMont

and the bid may well have put Salt Lake's candidacy at risk as well, had the USOC known.

Continuing the story, the paper said,

> LaMont's tax problems capped nearly a full day of testimony in the trial of Welch and Johnson [the leaders of the Salt Lake City Bid Committee] on charges of conspiracy, fraud, and racketeering in connection with the more than $1 million in cash and gifts handed out to International Olympic Committee members during their bid.

> The pair hired LaMont in 1989 to help Salt Lake City win the votes of the USOC as the country's candidate for the 1998 Winter Games.

There is no indication that the United States Olympic Committee ever knew that one of their key employees was being paid by Salt Lake City's Bid Committee to win votes for Salt Lake in their competition against Anchorage. Or that he was turning over information about Anchorage's bid to the Salt Lake City Bid Committee. In fact, LaMont had said to Welch or Johnson that he would "be fired" if the USOC ever found out what he was doing and he wanted assurance that if that happened he would get a job, at least at a vice president level, with their Bid Committee. When this relationship was discovered the USOC fired LaMont.

Four of the charges against Welch and Johnson were dropped when Federal Judge Dave Sam found that the Utah commercial bribery statute is, "ambiguous and unconstitutionally vague as applied in this case." Ultimately all the charges were dropped.

As I read letters to the editors of the Salt Lake papers about the scandal when it was happening, the ones that I remember were the ones that said the charges should be dropped because it was a "victimless crime." That was not accurate. There was a victim. It was the people of Alaska who spent nearly $6 million and tens of thousands of hours of volunteer work over five years only to lose unfairly.

Although Anchorage lost, we competed with decency, honesty, and honor. For that reason, all those who gave so much time and effort to bring the Olympics to Alaska should be proud of their contribution for the rest of their lives.

Since then major reorganizations have taken place with the USOC and the IOC and the Olympic movement is stronger and better as a result. In Salt Lake City, Mitt Romney was hired to repair the mess left by the previous leadership. He did a magnificent job of turning around the organization and creating a very successful Olympic Winter Games. Bill Marriott of the Marriott Hotel chain said that Mitt Romney brought the Salt Lake Games "… from a big mess to a big success." Salt Lake City, the USOC, and America have much to be proud of by the way Salt Lake City recovered from their scandal-ridden bid and hosted a successful games.

If you lose, lose with honor so at least honor survives.

—Rick Mystrom

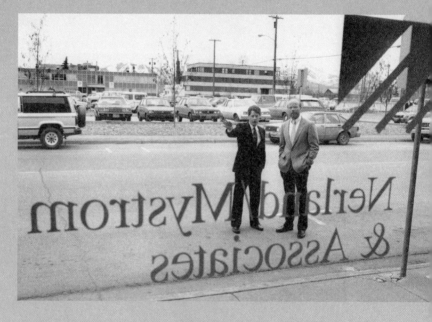

On March 1st, 1990 I concluded the sale of my advertising agency to Rick Nerland. Here we're viewing the new name on the window "Nerland Mystrom" which he kept for a year then changed the name to the Nerland Agency. It's now celebrating its 38th consecutive year of profitability—18 years under my ownership and 20 years under Rick Nerland's ownership.

Chapter 12

"The End of a Golden Era"

The day the Anchorage Bid Committee returned to Anchorage on June 16, 1989, from the USOC meeting in Des Moines, the *Anchorage Times* ran a banner headline proclaiming the loss to Salt Lake City "The End of a Golden Era."

In many ways that was true. During the depressed economy in Alaska in the late 1980s, the newspapers wrote daily of business closings, bankruptcies, home foreclosures, bank closings, and outmigration of residents. Only the tourism industry seemed to be prospering largely because—according to the visitor industry leaders—of the five years of extensive worldwide newspaper, TV, and magazine coverage of Alaska's Olympic bids.

But now Anchorage's Olympic bids were over—at least for the foreseeable future. Now, almost 24 years later, I see the possibilities of Anchorage hosting the Olympic Winter Games in 2026. But in July 1989 after the tie vote with Salt Lake was broken with the deciding vote being cast by then president of the USOC, Bob Helmick, it became a time of reflection for me. After five years as a full-time volunteer leading Anchorage's and America's Winter Olympic bids, would I feel satisfied or even motivated to settle in running my advertising agency? If not, what other options appealed to me?

At that time none of us on the Anchorage Organizing Committee had any idea that the leadership of the Salt Lake City Bid Committee would, years later, be facing federal accusations of bribery and corruption stemming from their competition with Anchorage. The resulting scandal would cause a number of IOC members to resign or be removed from their positions and cause a major restructuring of the United States Olympic Committee. But in 1989 we thought, naively as it turned out, that we had been beaten fairly in a close fight.

By July 1989 I had lived in Anchorage for a little more than 17 years. Mary and I were raising our family here. We were both involved in our kids' schools and their extracurricular activities as well as many community service organizations. I owned two businesses in Anchorage and had served for six years on the Anchorage Assembly, but nothing cemented my love for Anchorage like the reaction of our citizens following our loss to Salt Lake City.

From letters to the editors, to editorials in newspapers statewide, to resolutions of appreciation from organizations from Nome to Ketchikan, to everyday citizens on the streets, expressions of pride flooded in. As our committee members went back about their daily business, they were stopped dozens of time a day by people expressing their gratitude for bringing a sense of community pride to our city and state. As we got back to the business of closing down our organization, the members of the board of directors shared the comments they had received from people on the street, the word *proud* kept coming up time after time. "You made us proud," "I've never been so proud to be an Alaskan," "We're so proud of how you represented our city."

Among the hundreds of letters received after the loss, this one from Paul Davis, a longtime friend and prominent Alaskan trial lawyer, seemed to well represent many of the sentiments expressed by so many Alaskans.

Dear Rick,

I'd like to thank you on behalf of myself, Suzanne, and my family for all of the work that you and Mary put into the Anchorage bid for the Winter Olympics. I know that you must be profoundly disappointed in the vote at Des Moines. We share your disappointment. But our disappointment is limited only to the vote. You, Mary, and the other AOC leaders gave of yourselves far more than any of us had the right to ask.… Thank you for all your effort and the spirit that you helped create. Although this particular dream may not be reached, at least for now, the spirit that was created will birth other dreams. I am convinced that without your leadership we may not have achieved the reawakening of the Alaskan spirit that we need so desperately in these times.

Sincerely
Paul Davis

But from my point of view that pride was reciprocal. Hundreds of citizens made big financial or time commitments to the bid. Thousands took part in some way and well over 100,000 Alaskans donated their money to our bid effort. And no one came up to me, or as far as I know to any other member of the Bid Committee, and said, "What a waste of time," or "We never had a chance anyway." No one, not one person said that. Some may have felt it, but Alaskans in general are respectful of those who pursue dreams with or without success. I have never felt prouder of my hometown than I did then.

Selling My Advertising Agency

It was during those months after the bid that I first thought seriously about running for mayor of Anchorage. But in the immediate future all of us on the Anchorage Organizing Committee had families and/or businesses to attend to and lives to live outside the Olympic movement.

I had two businesses that had survived well despite my many absences. One was my apartment business, American Multiplex, managed by a bright, young, multitalented guy named David Borer. It was recovering from Alaska's economic devastation resulting from the dramatic drop in the price of oil beginning early in 1986. I hadn't seen the possibility of the price of oil collapsing but I did see some worrisome overbuilding in 1985. As a result, I had sold many of our properties before Alaska's real estate crash of 1986–87 and had started buying back in 1988, but the company was not yet big enough to support my family or to provide a continuation of the adrenaline-filled challenges and excitement I had lived through the preceding five years.

The other business was my advertising agency. Under the exceptional leadership of Linda Boochever, it had continued to grow and remain profitable. But after being a player on the worldwide Olympic stage, I felt my enthusiasm for running the company waning. Years before, I had run up the stairs two at a time on Monday mornings, excited about the coming week, but now I didn't feel that heart-pumping rush on Monday mornings. I felt okay about running the company but success demands more than "okay." After many discussions with Mary, I decided to sell the ad agency and run for mayor.

I wanted to sell the business to someone honest, smart, committed to Alaska, and capable of growing the company and serving our clients well. I knew just the right person: Rick Nerland. Rick had done a marvelous job as executive director of the Anchorage Organizing Committee. He was a fourth-generation Alaskan and very well known throughout the state, and with our Olympic bid over, he was now looking at a new career path. Within a short period of time, Rick bought a minority interest in the company. On March 1, 1990 Rick became the sole owner. On March 14 I filed to run for mayor of Anchorage.

My First Run for Mayor

The first term of the incumbent mayor, Tom Fink, was coming to an end. That term—Anchorage's mayoral terms are three years—took place during the worst economic depression in Anchorage's 75-year history. By the time Mayor Fink took office in 1987, Anchorage was in an economic recession. Nearly a dozen financial institutions would fail during this time and thousands of homes and condos were foreclosed by lenders or deserted by owners—a tough time for our citizens and a tough time to be mayor.

Now, 25 years later I realize that Mayor Fink and his unwavering conservative philosophy were well suited to the time. He had to cut government and he did. But at the time, the *Anchorage Daily News*, a liberal but very readable newspaper, with a fast-growing and large circulation, was merciless in their attacks on him for taking on the unions and reducing services to a broad range of tax receivers and nonprofit social service agencies.

The Most Creative Political Advertising Ads in America

Mayor Tom Fink was my main opponent in the race. But another well-known political figure entered the race, the former mayor of Fairbanks and former lieutenant governor, Red Boucher, a Democrat.

To call the ad campaign, "the most creative political advertising campaign in America" may sound a little vain and exaggerated, but it's neither. It's not vain because, unfortunately, it wasn't my campaign, it was my opponent's. It's not an exaggeration because the campaign was indeed selected by the American Association of Political Consultants as America's best political newspaper campaign for the 1988–1990 election years. The campaign was created by Dave Dittman of Dittman Research and Communication.

Dittman's strategy and execution were brilliant. As he explained his strategy to me when I was researching this book—more than 20 years after the actual campaign— "You were too popular and I didn't want Tom to have to run against you. I decided he should run against the *Anchorage Daily News* instead."

Tom's campaign did just that. His first ad had a photo of Mayor Fink hitchhiking out of town with his foot resting on an overstuffed suitcase. The headline said "If I believed everything the *Anchorage Daily News* said about me, I'd leave town." Each ad from that point on made fun of the *Daily News* and himself and said little about me.

We responded with some creative ads ourselves, but the Dittman strategy defined the campaign and we were definitely on the defensive. Although I started out with a significant lead, Mayor Fink gradually gained on me throughout the campaign until on election day we finished in a virtual tie, each of us just shy of the required 40 percent of Anchorage voters needed for an outright victory. The former lieutenant governor, Red Boucher, received about 20 percent so Mayor Fink and I went to a runoff.

During that campaign I got my introduction to the NEA, the National Education Association. Each of us three candidates were asked to make a presentation to a key NEA committee with one candidate to get their endorsement and theoretically the support and votes of the teachers and employees of the Anchorage School District, one of the largest school districts in America.

Before Red Boucher was eliminated from the race, I didn't expect to get the support of the various Municipality of Anchorage employees' unions because during my six years on the Anchorage Assembly I was one of the key leaders on a tax cap—which the unions, of course, didn't like. And I had worked to reduce the extraordinarily generous vacation that accrued very quickly to city employees.

But the NEA? Maybe. My wife and I had been what Jim Graham, our kids' elementary school principal, called, "our go-to parents." From elementary school through high school we were the ones the principals called on to organize, lead, or do whatever they needed. We were both PTA leaders and Mary worked for eight years along with Susan Sullivan and Pam Brady, two other very committed parents, to get a science wing built for West Anchorage High School.

I knew Mayor Fink wouldn't be endorsed by the NEA and during one of the early presentations Red Boucher, who had not lived in Anchorage long, candidly admitted he had not actually been in any Anchorage schools but said he intended to visit some during the campaign. I thought my chances of an endorsement were pretty good—a 15-year school volunteer vs. someone who actually had not even been in an Anchorage school. I certainly had demonstrated support of education in Anchorage and after all, this was the National *Education* Association.

How naïve of me! They endorsed Red Boucher, who committed to support what the union wanted. I don't think it made much difference. Even with his commitment from most of the unions, he still got only 20 percent of the vote.

Mayor Fink narrowly beat me in the runoff. I left that race disappointed, of course, but much better prepared for the next mayor's race in just over three years. I also left that campaign with the feeling that Tom Fink was the most honorable man I ever ran against and still hold that opinion today.

But before I ran again for mayor, I endured an injury that tested whether my health and circulation as a 30-year diabetic were robust enough to save one or both of my legs.

A shipwreck at sea can ruin a whole day.

—Doug Jackson (1967)

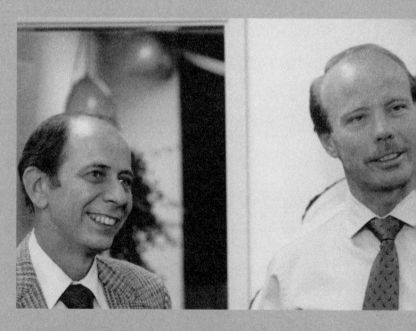

Dave Baumeister, president of the Anchorage Organizing Committee, my partner in the Olympic movement, and my lifelong friend; with me at the tenth anniversary celebration of Mystrom Advertising.

Chapter 13

Good Diabetic Health Saves My Legs

Anchorage's Olympic bid ended officially on June 4, 1989 with Salt Lake City's bribery-tainted, whisker-thin win over Anchorage. Less than two years later, another loss delivered a body blow to the Anchorage Bid Committee members and to thousands of Anchorage citizens and people throughout Alaska. Dave Baumeister, the president of the Anchorage Organizing Committee and one of my closest friends, died following a recurrence of non-Hodgkins lymphoma. Dave died on February 14, 1991, leaving his wife, Peggy, and three teenage children—John, now a firefighter in Anchorage; Laura, a teacher in Portland; and Sarah, a teacher in Anchorage. Dave would have been so proud of them. Peggy is.

On Memorial Day of that year four of Dave's closest friends—Bill McKay, Tom Tierney, Wilbur O'Brian, and I—flew to Seward, Alaska to spread Dave's ashes in Resurrection Bay. Dave often fished for silver salmon in Resurrection Bay with friends and clients. His company kept a beautiful yacht in a slip at the Seward marina and we planned to go out on her. My recollection is that she was a 65-foot Hatteras capable of sleeping eight comfortably. The four of us boarded the ship the afternoon before Memorial Day and motored out a few hours to one of Dave's favorite coves.

It was a beautiful, calm evening in a spectacular setting. We set some shrimp pots, fixed a decent dinner, and sat out on the deck regaling each other with Dave Baumeister stories. After lots of stories, shared memories, and more than a few drinks, we decided to spread Dave's ashes the next morning.

Our plan was to raise the shrimp pots in the morning, stow the gear, then slowly circle the cove while spreading Dave's ashes. Then we'd head to a good halibut-fishing area. We planned to cook the shrimp for lunch and bring the halibut we expected to catch home to Anchorage. That was our plan.

The next morning dawned sunny and calm—a little crisp but not cold enough to prompt wearing any more than a sweater on deck. After a couple of cups of coffee to chase the morning chill, we pulled the shrimp pots and found just enough for a good meal for the four of us plus the captain and the deckhand. We stowed the shrimp pots and put the shrimp in a 5-gallon aluminum stockpot and put it on the stovetop in the galley.

As we got underway, moving around the peaceful cove so slowly we hardly created a wake, the four of us stepped out onto the platform off the stern of the ship for an impromptu ceremony. We each took part in the spreading of Dave's ashes into the waters of the cove and each shared memories and respect for our beloved friend. The process was heavy on love, light on religion, and sprinkled with a modicum of irreverence. Dave would have liked it.

Everything Changes in an Instant

As we headed toward the halibut-fishing area we pretty much agreed that none of us could recall seeing Resurrection Bay so calm. Perhaps it was that smooth motion and the steady hand of the captain that gave us so much confidence that we didn't think about how foolish it was to have the shrimp boiling on the galley stove as we were underway.

Tom and Bill were sitting at a table five steps from the galley, Wilbur was standing on the steps leading to the upper deck, and I was carrying a salad to the table. At the very instant when I passed in front of the boiling water we hit a submerged rock. I screamed as 5 gallons of boiling water hit me full on—from my upper thighs to my ankles. I frantically yanked at my boiling hot pants. I couldn't undo the clasps. Tom suddenly appeared before me. He fell to his knees and with an adrenaline-filled rip, tore my pants in two.

As Tom pulled the torn remnants off, I looked down. Much of the skin was gone from both thighs. My left leg from my knees down to my ankle was covered in blisters. My right leg was burned but no instant blisters appeared. The salon was in chaos with furniture askew. The ship bounced against the submerged rocks, slightly tilting, furniture flung around looking even more disjointed. Together, my three friends got me moved to a long sofa still in place.

Twenty years later Bill recalled, "We hit the first rock, the bow went up, then we hit again as the ship dropped. I remember Wilbur being knocked off the ladder and bruising his hip in the fall." Neither Tom nor Bill, who had been seated at the table, was injured.

Bill asked the key question. "If you start to have any diabetic-related problems should we give you insulin or food?" I told him "Food."

The safest action for emergency treatment of any diabetic who is apparently having problems is something sweet to eat or drink. In my experience almost all cases causing a sudden problem are related to *low* blood sugar. The solution is something sweet. In the rare event that a sudden problem is the result of high blood sugar, it's unlikely that additional food or sweets would do any further damage. A high blood sugar problem has probably been a while developing and would typically not come on suddenly.

The captain dashed past me heading below deck to see if the hull was breached. He glanced at me and exclaimed, "Oh, Rick!"

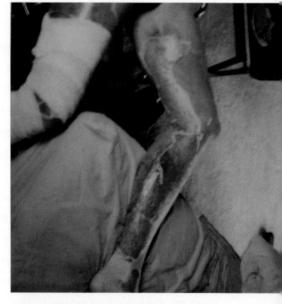

My legs approximately one week after the May 1991 boat accident out of Seward, Alaska.

in a tone that can only be described as coming from someone who deeply cared.

Tom stayed with me near the life raft while Bill and Wilbur, assuming we had breached the hull, squeezed into survival suits—flotation suits designed to keep users afloat and warm in cold Alaska waters. Tom later told me that the plan was for him to get into the life raft with me while the other guys in survival suits held on to the sides so we'd all stay together.

Upon striking the rocks, the captain had immediately sent out an SOS. By multiple strokes of luck, a chartered halibut-fishing boat was only about 15 minutes away. The boat, I found out later, was reputed to be the fastest halibut boat in Seward and even more fortunate was the fact that two of their on-board fishing clients were nurses from Providence Hospital in Anchorage.

As Bill told me later, "We lashed the two ships together and as we were trying to figure out how we were going to transfer you, a big, bald halibut guide who resembled Mr. Clean, only stronger, said 'Here's how we'll do it.' He picked you up and climbed over the railing with you in his arms." Actually, I'm glad I don't remember that.

What I do remember is being laid down on the floor of the boat and the two nurses comforting me and trying to keep me warm since my legs, without skin to hold heat in, were steaming from all the heat they were losing. The only medication on board was Tylenol. They gave me some. I don't know how many but if they had asked I would have suggested maybe 150. But they didn't ask. They put blankets over me and kept handing me glasses of hot water for me to drink in an effort to keep my temperature from dropping too fast.

Bill recalled that by the time I was in the rescue boat, a second, larger commercial boat had arrived on the scene. With that boat on site, Bill, Tom, and Wilbur felt the captain and crewman were out of danger and climbed into the boat I was on. They hung out on the back deck for the two-hour trip to Seward Harbor. I recall someone telling me that an ambulance would meet us at the dock to get me to the Seward Hospital and that a medevac plane from Anchorage with my wife on board would be in the air in moments to transfer me to Providence Hospital in Anchorage.

I don't remember much about the ride to Seward Harbor. I recall only talking with the nurses on board and the sirens going off as we entered the harbor. At the dock I was transferred to an ambulance and then to the Seward hospital.

In the emergency room at the hospital I was met by a team of medical personnel. After an examination of my legs, the lead doctor opined that the burns were not life-threatening. He also noted how high the burns reached up on my thighs and with a wry smile he said, "Good thing you're so tall." I knew immediately what he meant and managed a sincere smile. He also felt the pulse in my feet and declared I had great circulation in my lower extremities and that boded well for saving my legs. Then I remember a nurse inserting a morphine drip, which didn't make the pain go away but it seemed to move the pain out of my body and put it over in the corner of the room—a strange experience. My last memory there is of Mary just appearing and being at my side, where she always seemed to be in times of crisis.

In a short time I was in an ambulance again on my way to the Seward airport. There I was transferred to an Anchorage-based medevac plane which had delivered Mary to Seward and would bring us both back to Anchorage. In Anchorage I was transferred to a waiting ambulance to get me to Providence Hospital.

A medical team met me in the burn unit at Providence. I was immediately put in a sling and lowered into a tub of hot water that I recall had the word *lye* in bold letters on the tub. The lead team member told me that in order to minimize the potential for infection they would have to remove the dead skin from my legs. And since it was a scald, not a fire burn, they would have to shave my legs after they removed skin. Even with the morphine drip, having my legs shaved with no skin on them was a pretty rough experience.

The team then carefully bandaged both legs completely and got me settled in a room. Early the next morning Dr. Bonar was at my bedside. She had read the doctor's reports from Seward and from Providence and after checking the pulse in my feet she also said my strong pulse boded well for healing. But she couldn't make any assessment of my chances of saving my leg or legs until the next changing of my dressings. The changing of the dressings turned out to be a nightmare of pain despite the care and gentle touches of the nurses. It had to be done twice a day for weeks, then once a day after that.

Dr. Bonar was back in my room later that night for the first changing of the dressing. She got a chance to see the burns for the first time and said she thought my legs would heal and amputation would not be an issue if I could avoid infection. We talked about my diabetic condition and the challenges I would have with blood sugar control during the healing process. She explained that the burn center would put me on a very high calorie diet—like 8,000 calories a day to provide the fuel to keep me warm and regrow my skin.

The challenge Dr. Bonar and I discussed was that with an 8,000-calorie-a-day diet I'd have huge rises in glucose, which would require more insulin than I had ever given myself on a daily basis. Combine that with no exercise and no activity that I could take part in and my insulin requirement would be huge. I could be giving myself about 100 units of insulin a day instead of my typical 30–35 units.

I immediately recognized the problem. Big swings are much harder to control than small swings. It's a lot easier to heat a cabin in Alaska with a potbellied stove to a consistent temperature if the outside temperature is 50 degrees and I want the inside to be 70 degrees than if it's minus 40 outside with the same goal of 70 degrees inside. In the first case, to warm the cabin 20 degrees, I'd build a small fire in the stove and as the logs started to burn down I'd put another log in. In this scenario, the inside cabin temperature might range from 65 to 75 degrees—a pretty small swing. In the second case, trying to warm the cabin from minus 40 to plus 70—a rise of 110 degrees, would require a big fire and a continual replenishing of logs. If I were too slow adding new logs the temperature would drop fast. The inside temperature could easily vary from 50 to 80 degrees. Under those circumstances, I would have a hard time controlling the temperature in the cabin.

I realized the same thing would hold with large amounts of food intake and large doses of insulin. My swings would be greater than with smaller amounts of food and less insulin. Instead of my more typical swings of maybe 60 mg/dl to 170 mg/dl, I could possibly be experiencing swings from 40 or lower to 300 or higher. Both Dr. Bonar and I realized the danger in swings of that magnitude—especially on the low side—and the vigilance it would require for me to moderate the swings.

This axiom holds true with insulin-dependent diabetics under normal circumstances also. The larger the swings, the more likely a dangerous low will occur—especially at night. To avoid this danger, eat dinner as early as possible and eat foods for dinner that require less insulin. Blood sugar control for Type 1 and Type 2 diabetics is covered in detail in my companion book, *The New Diabetic Lifestyle.*

I had to be aware of these dangers, but the unforgiving presence of pain dominated every hour in the weeks following the accident. The twice-daily changes of the dressings were dreadful and between the changes, I could only lie motionless on my back. Even putting a sheet on would cause great pain. During that time I entertained scores of my friends in my underwear. Fortunately, upon entering my room, no one laughed and no one left.

After only four days in the burn unit, the doctors felt I could go home and Mary could drive me back to the hospital daily for my dressing changes. When we arrived home, Mary wheeled me up our sidewalk to the entry to our house. As we entered the foyer and I looked at the large curving staircase leading up to our bedroom, I saw an 18-foot cliff, not the easily navigable staircase I had left a week before.

What Mary and I devised was to be known as the "butt climb" and "butt descent," depending upon whether I was going up or down the staircase. To get up the stairs, I'd start on the first floor with my back to the stairs, put both hands on the step above and lift my butt up one stair. I'd repeat that over and over until I finally reached the top. That became my method of travel upstairs, downstairs, and around the house for the next month. Although I had to do that for only a month, it gave me a lifelong empathy, admiration, and respect for those who have the courage and perseverance to deal with mobility disabilities much greater and more permanent than the ones I faced.

The third day home Mary got an urgent call from Dr. Bonar. She said a culture taken of my wound at my dressing change had shown a staph (staphylococcus) infection. She told Mary she had called in a prescription to the Carr's pharmacy about a mile from our home and said, "Get down there right away; get the prescription; then get Rick back to the hospital." Mary sent our daughter, Jen, down to Carr's and started getting me ready to go back to the hospital. We knew my leg was in imminent danger when Jen came running up the stairs with the medication in hand and said the pharmacist told her, "Take this and get it to your dad as fast as you can. Don't stop at the checkout counter. Run. Pay for it later. Go."

When we got to the hospital Mary wheeled me into the burn unit and the burn team immediately put me on an antibiotic drip. Fortunately, they got the infection controlled within a few days and I was headed home again. But my troubles weren't over.

The big swings in blood sugar that both Dr. Bonar and I feared did happen. About six weeks into my recovery, my blood sugar dropped to a point that triggered a seizure—that point is about 25 mg/dl. Mary was grocery shopping. I was home alone and lying in bed when the seizure happened.

I don't remember anything about it happening. I must have recovered on my own as my body pumped adrenaline in reaction to the seizure. Adrenaline triggers the release of stored glycogen from the liver, which is the body's mechanism to recover from the trauma of a seizure. I must have regained enough consciousness to call my sister-in-law, Midge Lindemann. She and her husband, Jim, lived less than a mile away and showed up in minutes after what Midge said was a "very confusing and disoriented phone call from Rick." As soon as they saw me, they knew what had happened and called 911. On her way back from the grocery store Mary saw the paramedics pull into our neighborhood and followed them right to our house.

Following their usual protocol, the paramedics put in a drip of DW 50 and transported me to the emergency room. My past seizures requiring trips to the emergency room had usually involved a one- or two-hour stay, by which time I was ready to leave. I typically didn't feel chipper and light-hearted when leaving but I would feel okay, and usually within another four hours I'd be back to normal. This time was different.

As I got up to leave, my back hurt so much I could hardly straighten up. At this stage of my burn recovery I could walk, but now my back kept me bent over. I was sure that with a night's rest my back pain would go away. I was wrong. The next morning, I couldn't straighten up at all. I walked so curled up that Mary, who is 5 feet 6 inches, towered about a foot above my head. She helped me out to the car and went to a chiropractor's office. The chiropractor was a softball buddy of mine and as soon as he saw us hobbling into his office, he said to Mary, "Do you know a good orthopedic surgeon?"

Mary got the name of a Dr. George Gates from a friend and called his office. We went in the next day to see him and to get an MRI (magnetic resonance image). It was a painful experience to try to straighten out enough to be inserted into the MRI machine, which reminded me of the iron lungs that kids with polio had to live in 40 years earlier. The MRI showed a severely ruptured disc that was apparently caused by the stress and compaction of the seizure. That was the first and only time a seizure caused an injury to me more serious than a black eye or a bruised forehead.

He set surgery for the following day at what seemed to be my second home, Providence Hospital. He recommended removing the ruptured disc material and not fusing the two vertebrae above and below the disc. He said the surrounding donut-shaped ligaments would gradually fill in and act like a disc. I had confidence in the logic of his recommendation and agreed to it.

The surgery could not have been more successful. Most of the pain was gone by the next day and the remainder slowly disappeared over the next year. That was 22 years ago and I haven't had any back pain since.

My legs also healed very well and have left me with no lingering problems and minimal scarring. That summer was the most inactive summer of my life but by the following summer, I was back to fishing, golfing, rafting, and playing softball.

The summer of 1991 was a hard one but thanks to a lot of folks and good diabetic health, I still have my legs and they work just fine. I offer my thanks to the captain of the halibut charter boat, whoever he is, to the nurses on board that boat, to the nurses in the burn unit at Providence Hospital for the wonderful care they gave me, and to Dr. Jeanne Bonar, my doctor and friend, whose vigilance, personal care, and quick action were instrumental in saving my legs. I also thank Dr. George Gates, whom I haven't seen for 20 years but whom I often think of when I swing a golf club or softball bat, or when I just bend down to pick up something.

I also owe a deep thanks to Tom Tierney and Bill McKay, two friends who gave me continual support during the healing. Bill was there to push me around the block in my wheelchair when I needed to get outside and Tom stopped by every day on his way home from work. I'll never forget their support. Most of all I want to thank Mary, who gave more support, encouragement, and help than I could have ever asked for throughout the hardest summer of my life.

Anchorage's Olympic bid was over. I had sold my advertising agency. My apartment business was growing but still relatively small. I was looking for a new challenge. I didn't find it. It found me.

All politics is local.

—Tip O' Neill

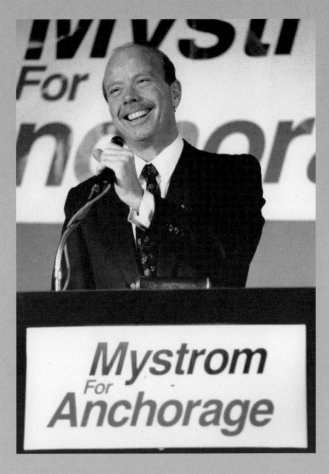

Speaking at one of my many campaign events while
running for mayor of Anchorage.

Chapter 14

Two Terms as Mayor of Anchorage

The Most Crowded Mayor's Race in Anchorage History

The 1990 mayor's race, which I lost in a runoff to the incumbent mayor, Tom Fink, had attracted only three well-known candidates, Mayor Fink, Red Boucher, a former lieutenant governor of Alaska, and me. But the 1993/94 mayor's race was a different story. Anchorage has a two-term limit for mayors. So with the current mayor unable to run, the seat was wide open.

As a result, everyone with name recognition, ambition, and the desire either to be mayor or to improve our city or both, filed for the office. The candidates were Mark Begich, an Anchorage assemblyman (currently the US senator from Alaska); Craig Campbell, chairman of the Anchorage Assembly; Virginia Collins, former Alaska state senator; Heather Flynn, Anchorage assemblywoman and former school board president; Jim Kubitz, Anchorage assemblyman; Joyce Murphy, a veterinarian and community activist; Pat Parnell, former Alaska state representative and father of our current governor, Sean Parnell; and me.

With that many candidates, it was clear none would get the 40 percent necessary to win without a runoff. Most knowledgeable observers felt that getting 20 percent of the vote would be all that was needed to get into a runoff. They were right. I led most of the six-month-long campaign with about 22 percent of likely voters supporting me, so during that whole campaign I was a target-rich environment for most of the other candidates. It was without a doubt the most grueling campaign I've ever experienced, six months with only a two- percentage-point lead doesn't give one much chance to pause and reflect. The campaign was more like act, react, and then act again.

After six months of campaigning and nearly a million dollars spent by the candidates, I ended up with 22 percent of the vote and Mark Begich, who had strong support from all five municipal employee unions, had 20 percent. The rest of the vote was split among the other candidates with Craig Campbell leading that pack with 17 percent.

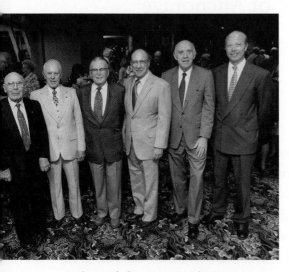

Anchorage's five surviving former mayors with me at an event honoring former mayor George Sharrock. *Left to right:* Bill Stolt, George Sharrock, Elmer Rasmuson, George M. Sullivan, Jack Roderick and me.

That set up a runoff between Begich and me. It was gloriously short, only about 30 days and I won by a large margin. The *Anchorage Daily News*, which had endorsed Begich, said "(Mystrom's) victory margin usually has the term *landslide* reserved for it." The *Times*, which endorsed me, said "… voter backlash against negative campaign ads was a factor in Mr. Mystrom's overwhelming victory." The newspapers called it a landslide or overwhelming. I just called it "satisfying."

Three years later I ran for reelection, won, and served a second three-year term. Former Mayor Fink filed to run against me at literally the last minute. He was my only opponent and ran a hard, issue-based campaign. I ended up winning by a significant majority—big enough to give me the mandate to continue pursuing my vision.

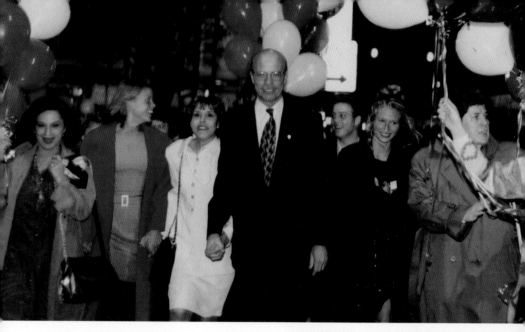

An Anchorage tradition, the candidates walk from their hotel campaign headquarters to election central at the Eagan Convention Center. Our daughter, Jen, in red coat; Mary and I, *center;* our son Rich to my left in back; Kathy Kingston, the city's director o f parks and recreation, in trench coat at right.

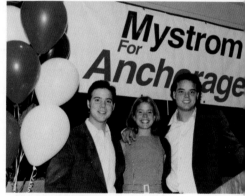

Our children, Rich, Jen, and Nick at my reelection campaign headquarters on April 15, 1997.

As I considered how to condense six years of 60-hour weeks into one chapter, I decided to focus on initiatives that were successful for Anchorage and which, I believe, can be adapted to other American cities and towns. In reading this chapter it's important to know that despite all the community-improving projects my administration undertook, we still kept every annual budget and consequently taxes far under the allowable tax caps imposed by the Anchorage Assembly 20 years earlier.

My administration left office with strong cash reserves in all our operating funds. We also left a general-fund reserve of $150 million. Of that money, $30 million could be spent by future mayors with the consent of the Anchorage Assembly and $120 million could be spent only by a vote of our citizens. Not surprisingly, the first $30 million was spent very quickly by my successor. The $120 million requiring voter approval has not been spent, and each year reduces property taxes based on its earnings.

My Vision for Anchorage

Throughout the six-month campaign for mayor, I talked about my vision to make Anchorage a safer, cleaner, more attractive city. But more than just explaining my goals, I explained why they were important. It's a message that I hope resonates with other mayors and civic leaders throughout America.

The basis for my vision was this. In each of the last three centuries, successful American cities had certain singular characteristics that determined their economic success.

In the 18th century, American cities had to have access to the Atlantic Ocean to be economically successful. They could be right on the ocean or on bays of the ocean or on rivers that had easy access to the ocean. This allowed for convenient export and import of goods to and from other countries and later to and from other states, and resulted in local growth and prosperity.

In the 19th century the most economically successful cities were those lucky enough or smart enough to have rail lines built near or through their cities—or even better, to have rail intersections in their cities. Those cities and towns prospered by being connected to the rest of America, especially the emerging west.

In the 20th century those cities which were able to accommodate the explosion of automobile ownership were the cities that grew and prospered the most. These were primarily cities of the American West, mostly young cities with more space for development of homes and freeways, the beneficiaries of the greatest migration in American history, the post–World War II migration from east to west. The ability to accommodate the automobile did not create the migration but without that ability, western cities would not have prospered.

So the obvious question for me as mayor of Anchorage was this: What is that singular dominant factor going to be for the 21st century?

Trying to project the most dominant factor for cities' success in the 21st century didn't take a lot of research. It just took an awareness of what was happening with the world's communication opportunities in the last decades of the 20th century and what that would mean to American cities. It was becoming more and more apparent that during the 21st century people would have much more freedom to choose where they wanted to live. They wouldn't necessarily have to live near their customers, near their suppliers, or near their company headquarters. More and more people could live where they chose, not where they had to. It became apparent to me that in the 21st century cities would prosper if they could create the quality of life that Americans wanted in their home city.

Quality of life would be that singular characteristic that would reap the most economic prosperity for cities in the 21st century. Quality of life as I saw it meant making Anchorage a great place to live, work, and play. As I often said in my speeches, the future belongs to those cities whose leaders understand that a good living, working, and playing environment will become an economic driver. I also knew that achieving a safer, cleaner, more attractive city was the starting point.

Although I recognized that economic success wasn't the only measure of a city's success, I also learned from experience that without a healthy economy it was difficult for a city to provide the amenities that created citizens' pride in their community. It was that pride, along with a vision for future improvement that would motivate citizens to follow a mayor's lead to make their city better. In fact, pride in our city was the component that would, in my mind, be the best measure of success or failure of my administration. Would the people of Anchorage be prouder of their city when I left office than when I came into office? If the answer was "Yes," we succeeded. If it was "No," we failed.

My goal of making Anchorage a safer, cleaner, more attractive city would go a long way toward creating the quality of life that would make Anchorage a more appealing place to live. I had a mandate from the voters who believed in that vision and elected me to make it happen. I knew the only way to make that vision a reality was with the support and involvement of our citizens. Now I had to get them to share in the effort to reach that goal.

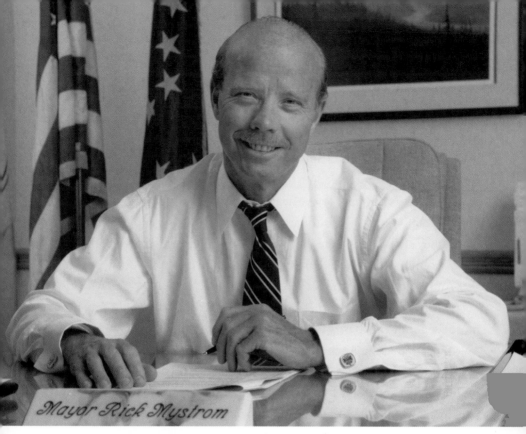

At my desk ready to get to work.

My First Week in Office

The path to developing my vision became much clearer at a lunch with Ken Thompson, then president of ARCO Alaska (now Conoco Phillips Alaska). Ken had invited me to lunch during my first week in office with the express purpose of sharing with me what he had learned in his business career about the difference between being a manager and being a leader.

"A leader," he told me over a halibut sandwich, "has only four primary responsibilities. The first responsibility is to develop a *vision*. The second is to develop a *strategy* to achieve that vision. The third is to line *up the people or resources* to make it happen and the fourth is to *motivate* all those involved." He followed up by saying, "If you do anything more than those four things you're managing, not leading. Let your managers do those things."

His advice was a key to my success as mayor and I'd recommend that advice to any big-city mayor. The mayors of smaller cities or towns often have to both lead and manage but the four principles still apply to the leadership portion of their jobs. Failure to appreciate this distinction between leaders and managers is one of the main reasons why small businesses don't become big businesses. Leaders of small businesses get too absorbed and involved in the day-to-day management functions and put their four primary functions, *vision, strategy, resources, and motivation* on the back burner. Business textbooks call it micromanaging. I call it losing the big picture.

I had another memorable meeting that first week in office. Dan Cuddy, president of First National Bank Alaska, came to my office to meet with me. Dan's one of the smartest people I know and I pay attention to what he says. But this time I hoped he was wrong. He said, "Mayor, I wanted to meet with you personally to tell you we're moving our bank's headquarters out of downtown Anchorage." I asked, "Why are you doing that, Dan?" He then said something I'll never forget. These were his exact words, "Downtown is dying and it'll be dead in five years." I responded, "Dan, give us a chance. I think we can revitalize downtown and bring it back." He said it was too late. The bank had already bought land in Midtown and would be under construction within a year. I thanked him for telling me personally, then moved *revitalizing downtown* up on my growing to-do list.

I also learned quickly about *asking* versus *telling.* Within the first couple of months in office, I *asked* our Parks and Recreation if they could convert a beautiful pond in west Anchorage, with the distinctly unappealing name of "Westchester Lagoon," into a natural outdoor skating rink in the winter. I got back a three-page memo explaining why it couldn't be done. By my second year in office, I realized I didn't have to ask them. I could *tell* them. It seems so simple but my style is more to get consensus from employees and peers rather than direct. But sometimes directing is better. I sketched out a drawing on a yellow piece of paper, sent it to the director of Parks and Recreation and said "Do this." They, of course, said, "Okay." They did a great job with the layout and execution and Westchester Lagoon has become a wonderfully active, Norman Rockwell-looking winter scene with hundreds of skaters of all ages on bright, sunny Alaskan winter days.

Building the Team to Execute the Vision

Very early in my administration, I put together what turned out to be a very effective leadership team. My executive committee developed our strategies and executed them through our department managers. This group would be a significant reason for our success over the next six years. It consisted of the following people:

Mary Hughes, a lifelong Alaskan and successful attorney. She was a whip-smart community leader with boundless energy. She not only brought clear and honest legal analysis and advice but more than that, she brought both creativity and common sense to our initiatives and played a huge role in our success. The city, as a perceived deep pocket, was—and still is—regularly getting sued by a variety of private citizens, special-interest groups, union members, and environmentalists. Mary's advice to me was beautifully simple: "The truth is always the best defense."

Larry Crawford had been the city manager under two previous administrations and brought an enormous amount of institutional knowledge and historical perspective to the executive committee. He brought us continuity when we thought that was appropriate. And he helped lead the city in new directions when that was our decision. (As an aside, Anchorage has a strong-mayor form of government, which means the mayor leads the city administration and has veto power over assembly action. Larry, as our city manager, did not report to the assembly or city council as a city manager would in a mayor-manager form of government. He reported directly to the mayor. Also, even though Anchorage is officially designated a *municipality,* for simplicity and clarity I use the term *city* in this book.)

Tom Tierney headed our human resources department and was our team's lead negotiator with multiple public-employee unions. Tom was smart and very tough. He had a personality that was a paradoxical combination of rock-hard cynicism and warm-hearted sincerity. Within six months he had solved Anchorage's biggest immediate financial threat by negotiating a $75 million decrease of the city's financial obligation with the Police and Fire Retiree Medical Funding Program. He achieved that by leading our team in negotiating a change from a defined benefit program to a defined contribution program.

Under Tom's leadership, we achieved agreements with four of the five largest municipal employees' unions. We were, however, in a stalemate with the Firefighters Union because we couldn't get their leadership to agree to random drug testing. We insisted they be subject to the city's random drug testing just as the police and most other city drivers were. Even though their members were driving the biggest and most expensive vehicles the city owned, their leader refused to accept random drug testing until the day after my successor was elected and the winner was not their candidate, Mark Begich. The day after Begich lost the election their union's attorney came into my office and said, "We'll sign."

Even though I had a city car, I wasn't required to have random drug testing since driving wasn't a big part of my job. Nevertheless, I voluntarily put myself into the police department testing pool and was in fact randomly tested for drugs during my terms in office.

George Vakalis headed our operating departments in the city. He was a hard-working, well-organized, by-the-book, on-the-ground leader. He had the loyalty of all the department heads because they knew he worked even harder than they did and he would always support them to me. I worked long hours—probably 60 hours most weeks—but George worked more than that. As an illustration of how hard our administrative leaders worked, one of our best and longest-term mayor's office staff persons, who worked under two mayors previous to me and two more following me, said shortly after her retirement that "no mayor's staff ever worked harder than Mayor Mystrom's staff did." It was a nice compliment from someone who had been working in the mayor's office more than 30 years.

Denise Burger completed our initial executive committee. She was my chief of staff and the catalyst for the whole office. She was organized, smart, and fun. Her staff employees put in long hours with no grumbling, regrets, or hesitation. In six years we had no personality problems or conflicts that so often detract from a work environment and interfere with the tasks at hand. Denise set the personality and tone for our office and it made my life as mayor much better. A big part of the credit for committed work of the staff and the success of our administration goes to Denise Burger.

Later I added *Elaine Christian* to the executive committee. Bright, young, and successful beyond her years, she had been the head of Covenant House, Alaska at the age of 25. She became our youngest department head when I hired her to head the Department of Health and Community Services at 28 years old. Following her success there, I brought her onto the executive committee during my second term and appointed her to the position of executive manager heading six staff departments.

My administration also started with a very competent and committed staff. Two longtime mayor's staff leaders, Nellan Budd and Judy Tymick, were indispensable. My appointed staff of Tim Rogers, Chuck Albrecht, and Pam Meistrel started us off strong, and Malcolm Roberts, Manny Wallace, Larry Anderson, and Valerie Hefner later added to our effectiveness.

First on my Agenda—A Safer City

Very early in our administration, we recognized the need for input from a wide variety of community leaders who would all have a role in reducing crime. To gather that input, we put together an extraordinary task force whose mission was to create what I called our "Community Action Plan on Crime" (CAP Crime). The goal I set for the plan completion was 120 days.

Among the leaders I called on to take part in this task force were the Anchorage chief of police and other key police officers, the heads of the Alaska State Troopers, the Alaska commissioner of Public Safety, the head of the Alaska Department of Corrections, the agent in charge of the FBI in Alaska, prosecuting attorneys, defense attorneys, and judges from the district court, the superior court, and the Alaska Supreme Court, including the chief justice. I also called on the superintendent of schools and other community leaders. Everyone I called accepted the responsibility and committed to the goal of reducing crime in Anchorage— though many thought my goal of cutting crime in half in six years was unattainable. George Vakalis took the staff lead on this task force and did a superior job.

Within four months the group completed Anchorage's CAP Crime, which the International Association of Police Chiefs would later call the best crime-reduction plan in America.

The executive committee began executing the plan the week it was completed. Our chief of police at the time, Kevin O'Leary, and the deputy chief, Duane Udland, were instrumental in implementing the plan. Among the many initiatives they started were expanding foot patrols downtown, establishing bike patrols in three high-crime areas, starting our version of community policing, and initiating a sexual-assault response team. They also established a misdemeanor follow-up team based on the premise that by taking misdemeanors seriously—especially those committed by young people—we would lessen the likelihood of those young people committing more serious crimes later. Our police department also partnered with the FBI, State Troopers, and the U.S. Drug Enforcement Agency to create what would become a very successful "Safe Streets Task Force."

Another major action I initiated based on the recommendation of Chief O'Leary was to change the police shifts from four consecutive ten-hour days to five consecutive eight-hour days. The authority to make this change was clearly spelled out in the police union contract.

The police union obviously didn't like my decision. I understood that. Their members had three days off every week and when combined with very generous vacation time, it was a dream situation for them. But

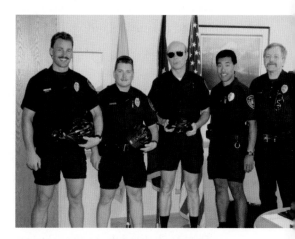

Going out to ride with Anchorage's bike patrol officers. I'm the skinny guy in the middle without a bulletproof vest. I guess they figured I was the most dispensable.

my goal was to make Anchorage safer and we were smack in the middle of what would become the highest crime year in Anchorage's history. My job was to do what was best for the citizens of Anchorage. As I saw it, this action was best. So I did it.

Switching to a five-8s schedule would increase the hours on the street per officer dramatically. With the previous four-10s schedule, the officers were on the street only eight hours each of the four days, then had an additional two hours back at headquarters. So Anchorage was getting only 32 hours a week on the street for each officer. With the five-8s' schedule, we immediately increased the hours on the street for each officer to 40. That meant a 33 percent increase in officers on the street at any given time. That single action was equivalent to adding 52 additional officers to the force at no additional cost.

In addition, the five consecutive eight-hour days made the shift scheduling much more effective. It's much less efficient to divide a 24-hour day into 10-hour shifts, with resulting overlap, than it is to use the standard eight-hour shift that most of America uses. That controversial change was a major step toward the biggest six-year reduction of crime in Anchorage's history.

Kevin O'Leary retired about a year after I became mayor and I quickly appointed Duane Udland as chief of police. He was an ideal candidate. His record was exemplary. He was smart, strong, and quietly charismatic and he was unanimously confirmed by the Anchorage Assembly. He turned out to be a great chief of police for Anchorage who was largely responsible for our dramatic reduction of crime.

We also made two of our higher-crime neighborhoods, Mountain View and Fairview, much less hospitable to drug traffickers and much more attractive to residents. We put 15 extra police officers in Mountain View. We initiated bike patrols in Fairview and we put a significant amount of capital project money into traffic calming in Fairview.

The idea behind the traffic calming was to make the neighborhood safer by slowing potential speeders, discouraging fast, pass-thru drug dealing, and generally bring attractiveness and pride to the neighborhood. To calm traffic we made many streets into cul-de-sacs, added curves, and built concrete landscaping planters designed and placed to slow traffic and add to neighborhood attractiveness. The traffic calming was enthusiastically supported by the home owners and resulted in lowering crime and increasing property values in Fairview.

Later, I authorized a major upgrade on 15th Avenue, the southern border of the Fairview neighborhood. We condemned some dilapidated, drug-infested, high-crime apartment buildings, widened the right of way and built one of the most attractive 12-block stretches of road in Anchorage. It stands today as an example of how major roads can and should look in our city.

We also cracked down on traffic scofflaws by publishing the names of people with outstanding traffic tickets in the daily newspaper. It was very effective and in the broad scheme of things, very cheap. Fortunately, I wasn't on the list.

To further make our streets less dangerous, the department focused on deterring different violations each week. One particular week we were focusing on speeding. One night during that week Mary and I, along with her sister, Midge, and her husband were returning from bowling. I was explaining how our police were cracking down on speeders. Just as I said that I glanced to my right and saw a police car parked on a side street and proudly said, "There's one now." Just as I said that he put on his lights and pulled in behind me. I looked at my speedometer and said, "Oh shoot," or words to that effect. By the time he pulled me over, he knew who he had stopped. He walked slowly up to my car, leaned into the window and said, "Mr. Mayor, now I'm in a terrible predicament." Before he explained any further, I stopped him and said, "No, you're not. If I was speeding you need to give me a ticket." I was speeding. He gave me a ticket and it was all okay.

Getting Rid of Graffiti and Junked Cars
—an Essential Part of a Safe City

To make the city clean and attractive, the first thing we needed to do was to get rid of the negatives: graffiti, junked cars, and trash. As Chief Udland directed the Anchorage Police Department's effort to make Anchorage safer, I instructed the Public Works Department to come up with a plan to get rid of graffiti and junked cars.

Under the leadership of George Vakalis, Jim Fero, and Joe Beauchamp we created and implemented two programs that made a huge difference in the attractiveness—and I believe the safety—of Anchorage. The first was *Graffiti Busters,* a program designed to get rid of graffiti in Anchorage. We established a Graffiti Busters hotline, which gave our citizens a vehicle to get involved. The Public Works Department promised to get rid of any graffiti reported on the Graffiti Busters hotline within one working day of the call. The public responded, big-time and so did the Public Works Department. By the time the vandals brought their friends by to brag about their desecration, it was gone—painted over with paint that matched the background—leaving no evidence it had ever been there. Once we took away the vandal's visual satisfaction, the graffiti began disappearing.

The word spread quickly to the public that if Graffiti Busters got a call, the graffiti would be gone within one workday. The more we kept our commitment to get rid of the graffiti, the more calls we got and the faster graffiti disappeared from our city. Unbelievably, within four months the graffiti was gone.

Operation Clean Sweep

The second program to rid the city of visual negatives was *Operation Clean Sweep*, a program that would, over the six years of my terms, remove more than 9,000 junked cars from the streets, vacant lots, and yards of Anchorage. We knew, with our commitment to clean up Anchorage, we could remove the junked, unlicensed cars on the streets but I wasn't so sure about junked cars in yards or on vacant lots.

Once again our city attorney, Mary Hughes, came through. She opined that with sufficient notice and sufficient opportunity to correct, we could indeed remove junked cars from private property. That's exactly how we acted. Our code enforcement people placed a fluorescent red notice on the cars which gave the "notice to correct" date and explained that if that condition were not met we would tow the vehicle and fine the owner $35 for the towing fee.

What happened next was something no one anticipated. As our city employees were putting the notice on the windshields of the junk cars, the owners often came out as asked what was going on. When it was explained that if they didn't correct the problem, we would tow their car and assess a $35 fine, the most common reaction was, "You mean you'll get rid of this piece of junk and only charge me $35?" When the city employee said, "Yup, that's essentially what we'll do," the typical reaction was for the owner to reach for his wallet and pay on the spot. With a receipt in hand the owner walked away happy and the car was removed within two weeks.

Getting rid of the trash was easier for us in the mayor's office because the Anchorage Chamber of Commerce had taken the lead on cleaning up Anchorage for decades. I just committed to doing everything I could to rally citizens to help the Chamber in their cleanup program.

Making a City Attractive Is More Than Getting Rid of the Negatives

Then I began the equally important task of getting Anchorage's businesses and citizens involved in making our community not just cleaner but more attractive. To get citizen buy-in we needed a goal and vision to work toward. The "City of Lights and Flowers" was my theme and our city loved it. With the well-deserved rough and rowdy image of Anchorage in the 1950s, '60s, and '70s, "Lights and Flowers" seemed almost un-Alaskan. But that theme counteracted the two negatives I often heard about Anchorage when I visited cities around the United States: too dark and too cold. Lights were a response to the dark perception and flowers a response to the cold perception. But more important, it was a theme that allowed all citizens so inclined to take part in making Anchorage more attractive in winter and summer.

The Anchorage Chamber had been working on a winter-lights program for years but without the initiative and clout of the mayor's office behind them, it was languishing. I made lights and flowers a central theme of the dozen or so speeches I was making every month during my first year.

Success beyond my most optimistic expectations started almost immediately. Under the creative and aggressive leadership of Kathy Kingston, my director of Parks and Beautification, local businesses donated over $450,000 to start the beautification of Anchorage. With that financial jump-start our summer employees created some of the most beautiful public floral displays in the United States. At the same time thousands of volunteers began cleaning up and beautifying their property. Sales at greenhouses and gardening supply stores blossomed in the spring and summer as people took more pride in how their yards and flower gardens looked. In the winter, home supply and lighting stores couldn't order decorative lights fast enough to keep up with demand. I recall walking into a Lowe's store and seeing a large sign saying "Out of decorative outdoor lights. We're flying more in. Come back tomorrow."

Competitions, sponsored by businesses, for the most beautiful home floral displays became part of summer in Anchorage. And in the winter, home and business light displays brought involvement, pride, and a sparkling festive look to our fast improving city. Anchorage was more attractive and its citizens were a lot prouder. A neighbor, Elizabeth Hickerson, whom I knew only casually then but whom I later came to regard highly, exclaimed that those first two years in Anchorage were like the scene in *The Wizard of Oz* where the land of Oz, "… went from black and white to Technicolor." Anchorage was definitely becoming much more colorful in the summer and brighter and cheerier in the winter.

By the end of our first year in office, the change in Anchorage was apparent. By the end of our second year, the change was dramatic. Anchorage was evolving from a gangling teen-ager of a city—with all the typical, early-pubescent blemishes—to a young adult in the world of American cities. Though it's very hard to measure, I do believe that cleaning up our city did contribute to reducing crime. I know for a fact—based on polling—that it did contribute to increased pride in our city.

In retrospect, I now realize that being a Republican made it easier to gain support for the lights, flowers, and beautification part of my agenda. If a Democrat had started out with my same beautification goals, he or she would likely have been met with skepticism reserved for "just another tree-hugging Democrat." The reverse also holds true. If a Democrat talks about cutting or limiting government, the media and the public will pay more attention than if that same action comes from "just another cost-cutting Republican."

Revitalizing Downtown Anchorage

The comment by Dan Cuddy during my first week in office that "downtown is dying and will be dead in five years," was never far from the front of my mind. I also knew that most successful American cities had vital downtowns which resulted in people living in those downtowns, not escaping by 5 p.m. every day. In Anchorage people were "escaping" downtown after work—and for good reason. The feel of the city changed after 5 p.m. and why wouldn't it? Downtown wasn't clean or attractive—or safe at night. It had a limited number of nice restaurants, mostly congregated on the far west end and it wasn't very comfortable to walk around downtown in the evening or later.

I knew what my vision for downtown was: a safe, clean, attractive downtown, but even after four months in office, I wasn't sure how I could get there. The police department was starting downtown bike patrols and foot patrols but that was just a small start to making downtown more vital. The real answer came to me at the first Conference of Northern Mayors I attended a few months after I started my first term. It was hosted by Mayor Sue Thompson of Winnipeg, Manitoba.

During the conference, Mayor Thompson hosted a dozen or so mayors for a tour of Winnipeg. It was a dreary, dark, late fall evening with no snow yet to offset the darkness with its white reflection. As we rode slowly down a dark, nearly deserted street, Mayor Thompson pointed out what she called "an oasis of light," a few blocks ahead. I recall it as a two- to four-block area that she called a "Business Improvement District." It was indeed an oasis of activity amid the dreary and inactive surrounding area. People were on the streets, in the stores and restaurants, and appeared genuinely happy and active.

We passed out of that area into more darkness and inactivity until we reached another oasis of brightness, another Business Improvement District, with more activity, more people, and a general appearance of prosperity and good feeling. By the time we passed through the fourth Business Improvement District, I realized I had found the solution to Anchorage's morose, unwelcoming, and somewhat depressed downtown.

Soon after my return from the conference I convened a committee of downtown business leaders to address the concept of an Anchorage downtown business improvement district. Under the leadership of Larry Cash, the head of a large architectural firm headquartered downtown and Chris Anderson, chairman of the Anchorage Convention and Visitors Bureau, and Janet and David McCabe, downtown residents, I organized a committee to develop the concept, organize a plan, and make it happen. I added one concept to the model I had seen in Manitoba. That addition was the idea of *downtown ambassadors* who would help and direct tourists or residents and help act as the eyes and ears of our police department on safety issues downtown.

The concept was to make downtown Anchorage one big business improvement district, over 100 square blocks. Since the city was the only body that could create and collect a property tax, our intent was to initiate a small raise in property taxes (an assessment) for those properties within the district. The city would collect the taxes, then return 100 percent of the money collected to a corporation to be created. That corporation could spend the money only on downtown improvements within the assessment area. To authorize the creation of the business improvement district, the committee and I needed the support of more than 50 percent of the property ownership within the district. To get that support we met two nights a week for six weeks to assign contacts and then met with downtown property owners during the day. Once we reached comfortably more than the 50 percent level of support, we began the legal and political process to make it happen.

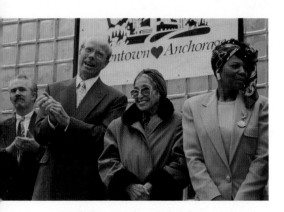

With Rosa Parks, civil rights icon, at one of many events celebrating the revival of downtown Anchorage. At left is Larry Cash, leader of the downtown revitalization movement, who gave a touching speech honoring Rosa Parks and her impact on America.

Once the concept was approved by the assembly, a corporation called the Anchorage Downtown Partnership (ADP) was created whose mission was to provide clean, safe, and vital services throughout the downtown improvement district (DID), provide marketing and event promotion throughout the DID, and serve as an advocate for the business and property owners within the DID on issues affecting downtown. The assessment now provides between 50 and 60 percent of the total budget for ADP annually, while nonassessment revenue comes from membership fees, sponsorships, contracts, and grants.

In addition to making downtown much cleaner and more attractive, the Downtown Partnership has brought a sense of pride and confidence in downtown Anchorage that has resulted in many new businesses, restaurants, and residents living downtown. Our new, more vibrant downtown has also contributed greatly to the increase in value of homes in the adjacent neighborhoods of South Addition, Inlet View, and Bootleggers Cove, all within walking distance of downtown. Downtown Anchorage is now the healthy, vital heart of our city.

A View from the Roof of Anchorage's Historic City Hall

As part of revitalizing downtown, I negotiated with the Anchorage Convention and Visitors Bureau to get them to renovate our 80-year-old historic Anchorage City Hall. The mostly privately supported Anchorage Convention and Visitors Bureau paid for the renovation and the city leased it to them at a discounted rate.

One Sunday morning during the construction, Mary and I were having breakfast across the street at the Downtown Deli. As we finished breakfast, I suggested we check out the renovation progress. The front door was unlocked and we walked into the vacant, under-construction building. As we were touring the second floor of the construction site, Mary noticed a stairway going up farther with a door at the top. She asked where that went. I said, "I don't know. Let's find out." We walked up and stepped outside onto the roof. As soon as I heard the door close behind us I murmured, "Uh oh, I bet it's locked." I was right. It was locked. We were locked out on the roof of the old city hall on a Sunday morning before the days of cell phones. No other way down and no way to climb down as far as I could tell.

We saw only a few early-morning tourists on the street within the three blocks in our sight. One group of four was about a half block away. I yelled out to them and motioned them toward us. When they got just below us, I shouted to them, "I'm the mayor. My wife and I are locked out on the roof of city hall. Can you open the roof door and let us out?" They smiled, responded positively, and walked into the building to look for the uncooperative door. But 15 seconds later they reappeared, pointed their video camera at me and said, "Excuse us, but would you say that again to our camera?"

Given my compromised situation, I repeated my plea to the camera and again asked for their help getting us off the roof. Satisfied and enjoying the whole episode, they again walked into the building. Another 15 seconds and they appeared below us again. They all looked up at me with a look that said, "Are we having fun or what?" Then they asked the watershed question, "Are you a Democrat or a Republican?" I said Republican. With a disconsolate look they collectively said, "Oh." But in the spirit of bipartisanship that is sometimes absent today, they did open the door and let us out.

Three More Good Ideas for American Cities to Consider

Three other programs I started as mayor are certainly worthy of consideration for adoption by other American cities. The first, *Good News, Great Kids,* was conceived to acknowledge and reward the community achievements of some of our high school students. The second, *Parent Networks,* was started to head off trouble among high school students before it developed. The third program, *BridgeBuilders,* was designed to build friendship and respect among all cultures and races in Anchorage.

Good News, Great Kids

This program was conceived during a discussion in our executive committee about all the negative news about youth that seemed to appear daily in crime reports and newspaper stories. It seemed like the only positive recognition for young people was found on the sports pages and on graduation days. The concept that evolved was to ask the principals of our public and private schools to identify young people who were making exceptional contributions to our community, to their classmates, or to any others who needed help. The kids didn't have to be honor students or student leaders. They just had to be kids who were helping others in the school or community. From the nominees, a committee selected 10 *great kids.*

At the recognition event conducted toward the end of each school year, every "great kid" is introduced and his or her story told by the current mayor of Anchorage. The student is brought forward for the *Great Kids* award. The unique part of this program is that the student recipients bring forward the one teacher they have chosen as the most influential and inspirational teacher in their lives. The recipient students then tell the story of the impact this teacher has had on each of their lives and present the teacher with their *most inspirational teacher award.* That portion of the program has become a heart-warming, tear-inspiring, pride-instilling element and will never be forgotten by student or teacher.

The program received a big boost late in my term from then president of the University of Alaska Mark Hamilton, who presented a $10,000 scholarship to each of the Great Kids honorees. The Good News, Great Kids continues today in its 18th year.

Parent Networks

Another simple but effective program we started was *Parent Networks*. At the start of each school year we worked with the school district to distribute brochures to parents of high-school-age kids, encouraging them to create a network of parents of their children's friends. Whether that network of parents consisted of as few as three parents or as many as 10, its purpose was the same: for all parents to exchange phone numbers and to agree that they wanted to be called if any of them saw or heard things that might be of concern. The issues could be unchaperoned parties, underage alcohol use, bullying, drug use, or any of a number of issues that create problematic behavior.

We encouraged the parents to get together for lunch or for coffee at the start of the school year to share contact information, then once or more during the year to assess how the kids seemed to be doing.

Very simply, Parent Networks puts parents on a more even communication footing with their high-school-age kids and gives parents the encouragement to call each other and not be considered intruding. It's a very simple program and does work.

BridgeBuilders

To add to our increasingly clean, attractive, and safe city, I wanted to ensure that no racial or cultural groups felt isolated within their chosen home city. I wanted to give all races and cultures access to political leaders *and* to the opportunity to become political leaders themselves. Anchorage, to the surprise of many, is a very culturally and racially diverse city. About 13 percent of our population is Asian, Pacific Islander, or Filipino; 9 percent is Alaska Native (Eskimo, Aleut, Tsimsian, Athabascan, Tlingit, or Haida); 11 percent is Hispanic; 6 percent is African American; and 12 percent is multiracial. The balance is Caucasian. In our 50,000-student Anchorage School District, the students enrolled in our English Language Learner's program speak 91 different languages at home.

Toward the end of my first term, Mary and I invited some African-American community leaders and some Caucasian community leaders to our home for dinner. The idea for that gathering came from an exchange of pulpits by two highly regarded Alaskan leaders of the faith communities. Dave Blievik, the pastor of the First Presbyterian Church, to which Mary and I belonged, and which had a predominantly Caucasian membership, exchanged pulpits one Sunday with Alonzo Patterson, the pastor of Shiloh Baptist Church, a predominantly African-American church.

The express topic for the dinner was improving relationships between blacks and whites in Anchorage, but it didn't take long for Pastor Patterson to say what should have been obvious to me—that it's "not just a black and white issue. It's an issue of all colors and races." In the three-hour discussion that followed, the concept of "BridgeBuilders of Anchorage" was born.

We started by inviting three couples from each of 15 different cultural and racial groups to an international potluck in our backyard. Each couple agreed to be matched, for one year, with a couple from a different racial or cultural group. During the course of their match each couple would invite the other couple to dinner with other friends from their cultural group. Each of the invitees would be asked to take part in the next annual BridgeBuilders international potluck dinner and be matched themselves with a couple from another culture. Five years later, at the last BridgeBuilders international potluck under my administration, we had over 400 citizens from 45 different cultural groups there to be matched for a year with couples and singles from other cultures and races.

Since then, BridgeBuilders has continued to grow and welcome Anchorage citizens of all races into its organization. Each year it hosts a *Meet the World* event at our museum to introduce residents to the cultures of the various birth countries of our citizens; it also continues to host the international potlucks, and an international gala recognizing leaders and volunteers from the various cultures and featuring dancers, singers, and entertainers from our many different cultures.

Many of our different cultural groups proudly take part in their new country's Fourth of July parade by building colorful floats reflecting their birth countries' traditions. For decades prior to my administration, Anchorage's Fourth of July parade had only a few high school bands, some military vehicles, some fire trucks, and very few spectators. Now the parade has hundreds of floats, thousands of participants, and spectators three deep along the downtown streets.

That parade is another example of how much I used Ken Thompson's advice: create the vision, develop the strategy, line up the right people to accomplish it, and motivate them. In this case, the right person was Tennys Owens, a smart, well-organized, hard-working community leader and art gallery owner. I met with Tennys one day on my way home from my Rotary meeting and shared with her my vision of a millennium celebration for our citizens as well as my desire to have a better July 4 parade. She was one of the Anchorage leaders who could make those things happen, but the key question was: Would she? She was already very much involved in other projects.

Two days later she called me and said "Yes." With the help of hundreds of volunteers she led the effort to create a six-month celebration starting with a spectacular New Year's Eve millennium event and ending with a reenergized Fourth of July parade.

BridgeBuilders also created the Pledge of Mutual Respect, a document distributed to schools throughout Anchorage in a citywide effort to get signatures of

The Pledge of Mutual Respect

We the people of Anchorage,
Alaska pledge to respect
one another;

Celebrating the differences that
make us unique; our customs,

Spiritual beliefs, cultures, colors,
dreams, and ancestral traditions.

Standing together, hand in hand,
young and old,

We affirm that through mutual
respect we can build

A stronger, more harmonious
community, a more unified
nation and

A better, safer world.

support from 50,000 Anchorage residents and have the pledge placed in classrooms throughout Anchorage.

This has been an extraordinarily successful program that I believe presents an opportunity for cities around the United States to adopt and add their own unique elements to. For our city it's been a friendship-building, pride-instilling, crime-reducing program that has made Anchorage a welcoming city to all races and cultures.

Although I started the program when I was mayor, the credit for continuing Bridgebuilders and bringing to our city all the goodwill the program creates belongs to those citizens from dozens of different cultures who continue to pursue the dream of Anchorage being a city without prejudice. My great respect and appreciation go to those from among those citizens who have given their energy, commitment, and leadership to the ideals of mutual respect among all races and cultures.

First and foremost are the indefatigable Malcolm and Cindy Roberts and the warmly articulate Elsa Sargento. They have been the backbone and strength of Bridgebuilders for well over a decade. Cofounders Alonzo Patterson, Dave Bleivik, Ted Moore, Paul Davis, and Mary Mystrom were all instrumental in conceiving and growing the program as well as composing the Pledge of Mutual Respect.

To the leaders of all the different cultural communities in Anchorage, thank you for bringing us all together multiple times every year to learn to respect each other's cultures and celebrate their beauty: *gracias, merci, mahalo, salamat po, arigato, havala, toda, spasibo, tack, kamsahamnida* and thank you for all you've done to make Anchorage a welcoming and safe city for us all.

In 2002, with BridgeBuilders as one of the three programs cited, Anchorage was recognized by the National Civic League as one of 10 All-American Cities. I highly recommend BridgeBuilders to other American cities. It has certainly instilled pride and mutual respect among the many races and cultures in Anchorage and has been effectively used here to diffuse or avoid potentially threatening situations.

Information about the program is accessible on the Internet by googling *BridgeBuilders of Anchorage.*

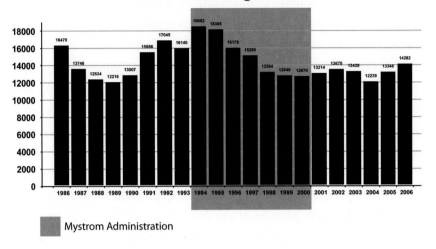

Crime in Anchorage 1986-2006

Mystrom Administration

The Result of the Combined Programs—A Big Crime Reduction

These initiatives I've described represent just a portion of the programs we implemented during my administration, but their effect on crime was dramatic. The year I took office did turn out to be the highest-crime year in Anchorage since the FBI began its standardized measurements of crime in the 100 largest American cities. That year we ranked 50th in terms of public safety of those 100 cities—dead center. By the time my administration left office six years later our city leaders, our city employees, and involved citizens had all contributed to the biggest six-year reduction in crime in Anchorage's history and one of the biggest crime reductions in America. In those six years we went from the 50th-safest city to the 16th-safest city in America and from the 8th-safest to the 2nd-safest among cities our size in America.

As I researched articles written about that era in Anchorage, I realized that I did not achieve all the goals I set for myself—specifically, I didn't reach my goal of cutting crime by 50 percent or my goal of making Anchorage the safest city of our size in America. But by setting our goals and expectations so high, we did achieve an extraordinary reduction in crime of about 40 percent and did become the second-safest city in America among cities our size.

To this day people still ask me how we brought crime down so dramatically and made Anchorage so much safer. The truth is I don't know exactly which of the programs or actions we initiated made the greatest contribution to the dramatic drop in crime. But together they worked. I can only surmise that ridding Anchorage of junked cars and graffiti, involving citizens in making the city cleaner and more attractive, opening our arms to people of all races, and improving the shifting and efficiency of our police department, and the many other programs we started all played a role in making Anchorage a much safer city.

All in all it was a productive and fulfilling two terms. I'm very proud of the results of our time in office. But more important, I left office feeling that our *citizens* were prouder of our city at the end of our administration than they were at the start of it. And that's what really counts. I'm now able to enjoy the only job in Anchorage that's better than mayor of Anchorage—and that's *former* mayor of Anchorage.

My Diabetic Experiences and Challenges as Mayor

I made it a point early in my first term to tell Denise Burger, my chief of staff, to always find time for me to meet with any young diabetics and/or their parents who needed encouragement. I met with many of them in the mayor's office and the meetings mostly seemed to be positive and encouraging. But with some young diabetics I sensed some anger and denial that I feared would make it more difficult for them to deal successfully with their challenges.

I did have one extreme low blood sugar (an event that required a trip to an emergency room) during the time I was mayor. It was the *last* extreme low blood sugar episode requiring emergency medical attention I have had.

In the fall of 1995, I took a short break from my mayoral duties and went to Seattle to play golf with Asa. We had three good days of golf including one round with my good friend, Bill McKay. Asa and I scheduled our last round on Saturday at a golf course not far from the airport. I was planning on flying home that Saturday evening after the round. I don't remember much about that round but my memory is clear that on the 18th hole as I walked up the fairway toward the last green I gave myself a small infusion with my insulin pump. Asa recalls that I measured my blood sugar. I don't recall that but I do remember the small infusion.

This was to be my first lesson about how many calories a round of golf burns even if you're using a cart. If you're walking and pushing or pulling a cart, of course you burn more and if you're walking and carrying your bag, you burn even more calories. I've also learned over the years that the calorie-burning process continues for about 30–60 minutes after the golf or other long activities end.

After we finished the round I remember Asa driving me to the airport where we found that my flight was going to be late departing. Instead of waiting at the airport, we decided to have dinner at the nearby Red Lion Hotel. By the time we got to the Red Lion, it was nearly 45 minutes since my infusion of insulin on the 18th hole. My blood sugar drop from that small infusion of insulin was compounded by the continuing "post-activity effect." By the time we walked into the lobby of the Red Lion, I recognized that my blood sugar was very low and told Asa.

I walked directly to the small convenience shop in the lobby, grabbed a candy bar, tore off the wrapper and started eating it. He had grabbed a soft drink and paid for both. As we walked out of the little shop back into the lobby, he later told me that I was "disoriented, pale, and wobbly." I started to fall. He caught me and held me up. He called to a bystander to slide a chair over and he sat me down in it. According to Asa, a guest came over and identified herself as a nurse and said they should lay me down on the floor. A physician then came over and felt for my pulse. The good news was he found one and he said it was strong.

Someone called an ambulance and within minutes it arrived. According to Asa, the first thing they did was take the batteries out of my pump to be sure no more insulin would go in. Then they measured my blood sugar, which he recalled was 28 mg/dl. Asa told this to me as I was doing research for this book and it remains the only time I've ever known exactly what my blood sugar was when I was unconscious. I've seen my blood sugar in the 30s and still been conscious and I vaguely recollect that I once measured a 27mg/dl while still conscious.

Asa recalled that I struggled against the paramedics as they strapped me to a gurney. As they put me into the ambulance he said I complained about cramps in my leg. Evidently, by that time, I was able to talk even though I was not aware of it.

Once again I was in a hospital emergency room as things started to clear up for me. The only part of the conversation I recall was the doctor asking me what I did in Anchorage. I told them I didn't know but that I used to be mayor. I heard the doctor repeat that to Asa outside the door and heard Asa say, "He still is." The next thing I heard from outside the room is the doctor telling someone, "We've got a mayor in there."

They kept me in the hospital only a short time—maybe an hour or so—then released me. I was worn out physically and emotionally as I usually am after one of these episodes. I called Mary to tell her what had happened and together we decided it would be best for me not to fly home that night but stay in a hotel near the airport and fly home the next day.

Mistakes That Caused This Episode

1. I don't recall measuring my blood sugar immediately prior to giving myself a small infusion of insulin. Avoid giving yourself insulin based on what you *think* your blood sugar is. Give yourself insulin only after you *know* what your blood sugar is.

2. I didn't understand the "continuation effect" of a long, calorie-burning activity. I've now realized that blood sugar continues to drop faster than normal for 30 to 60 minutes after a four- or five-hour physical activity. That drop combined with insulin going in (on board) can be dangerous. In this episode, having emergency glucose or candy might not have helped because I didn't realize my blood sugar was low until it was too late. I believe that the continuation effect plus the insulin going in were lowering my blood sugar so fast that by the time I felt it I was only a minute or so away from losing consciousness.

Two Other Low Blood Sugar Episodes

I did have two other low blood sugar episodes while I was mayor. Neither required a trip to the emergency room but both required help from other people.

One episode occurred during a mayors' conference in Kodiak, Alaska. I had just returned to my hotel from a short tour of Kodiak with the president of the Kodiak Chamber of Commerce, Andy Tierney. By the time I walked into the hotel lobby, I was disoriented. Chuck Greene, mayor of the Northwest Arctic Borough, took my arm and got me into my room. Chuck found my assistant, Pam Meistrel, and told her about my condition. By the time she got access to my room, I had evidently had a seizure and was in the recovery phase. She contacted Denise Burger and Mary and then stayed with me in the room that night until I was fully recovered.

The other episode happened in Amsterdam on a layover from Sweden heading back to Anchorage. I had made a presentation in Sweden promoting Anchorage as a site for the biannual International Conference of Northern Mayors. I was joined by members of the Anchorage Convention and Visitors Bureau and we were successful in being selected as the host city, which would be a good learning experience for Anchorage's leaders and an economic boost to our economy.

Larry Anderson, a staff member responsible for international trade and promotion, had accompanied me and coordinated the presentation. Larry and I had a 10-hour overnight layover in Amsterdam and stayed at a hotel near the Amsterdam Schiphol Airport. For dinner that night my main food was shrimp, with no carbohydrates. Once again I didn't pay enough attention to the small impact shrimp has on my blood sugar and I obviously gave myself too large an infusion of insulin. After eating I went up to my room to sleep.

The next thing I recall was wandering in a hotel hallway in my underwear, not knowing where I was or what happened. I ultimately found my way down to the lobby to ask the night clerks for help. They called an ambulance but by the time the medics arrived I had recovered sufficiently so that they felt no need to transport me to a hospital. While the paramedics were attending to me, the night manager checked out my hotel room.

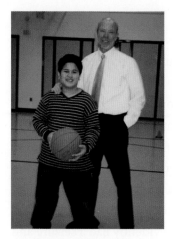

During my terms as mayor, I was a Big Brother to Josh Tofiano, a really great young kid who has become a successful, productive adult.

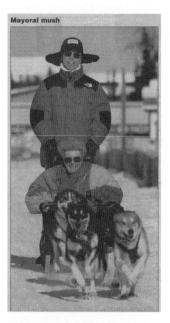

Taking my favorite American mayor, Beverly O'Neill, of Long Beach, California on a dogsled ride just prior to the 1998 Iditarod race.

Evidently I had had a seizure and thrown up in the room. They put me in a clean room and awakened Larry to gather my belongings from the old room. The next morning I was feeling, not chipper, but okay. Larry and I stayed on schedule for the 15-hour return flights to Anchorage.

Aside from the three issues I just discussed, I think the impact of having diabetes while running the city was pretty insignificant. My immediate staff was very much aware of the symptoms of low blood sugar that I might have and always carried some kind of sugar or glucose tablets in case I needed something to raise my blood sugar quickly. Most of the 5,000 or so city employees were at least vaguely aware of my condition so it was no surprise to anyone to see me testing my blood in meetings or prior to my giving one of my 100 or so speeches a year. During my two terms as mayor of Anchorage, being an insulin-dependent Type 1 diabetic never kept me from doing anything I wanted to do or needed to do as mayor.

The photos below represent some of the very enjoyable experiences I had as a physically active mayor.

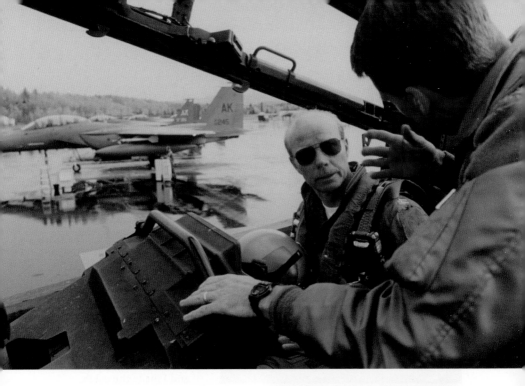

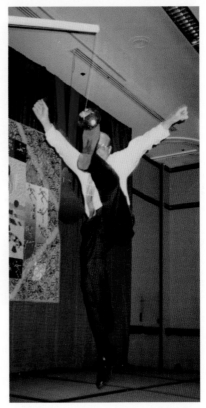

Top: One of Alaska's largest employers is Elmendorf Air Force Base. Here I'm getting final briefing from Captain Campbell just prior to an F-15 flight. His unforgettable instruction to me as we reached the training ground about 300 miles northwest of Anchorage and he handed the controls to me was, "Mr. Mayor, we've got 12,000 square miles and a $47-million-dollar video game. Have some fun."

Right: Not one to ever pass up an athletic challenge, even in a suit and tie, I agreed to attempt the one-foot-high kick at an opening event for the 1996 Arctic Winter Games. Here it looks like I've hit the target at about 6 feet 10 inches. The Arctic Winter Games record is 9 feet 8 inches.

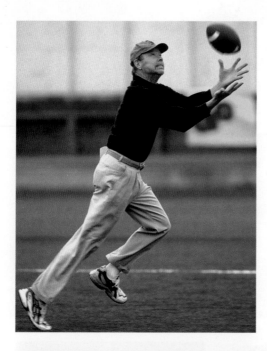

Instead of cutting a ribbon to dedicate the new artificial turf at the Anchorage Football Stadium, I decided to try to catch the first pass. Dimond High quarterback Jack Tomco threw a beautiful 50-yard spiral to my outstretched fingers at a full sprint on my 55-year-old legs. *Anchorage Daily News* photographer Erick Hill made the perfect photo and I made the catch.

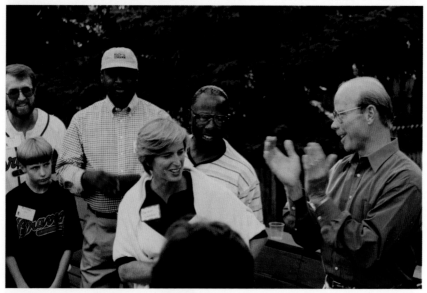

Summers in Alaska meant lots of outdoor events in our backyard during my terms as mayor. Here, Mary and I are hosting an event for Hank Aaron. Governor Christy Whitman of New Jersey, who had just finished a five-day bicycle trip in Alaska, stopped by. *Left to right:* longtime friend Rod Hill, his son Robbie, Bill Leavell, Governor Whitman, Hank Aaron, and me.

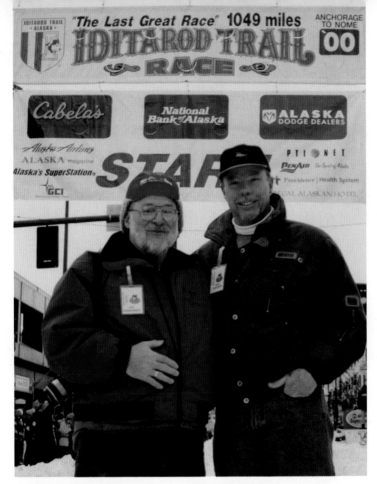

The Iditarod Sled Dog Race from Anchorage to Nome is billed as "The Last Great Race." Here I'm at the start in Anchorage with Nome legend and former mayor of Nome, Leo Rasmussen.

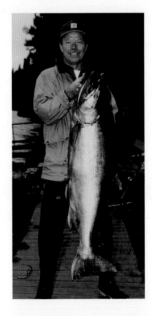

Sometimes I had to squeeze in the fun. On this day, I was up at 4 a.m., aboard a small plane to the Kenai River at 5 a.m., on the river at 6 a.m., on the dock with a 63-pound king salmon by 7 a.m., back in the office by 8:15 a.m. in time to give welcome comments to a company considering a move to Anchorage.

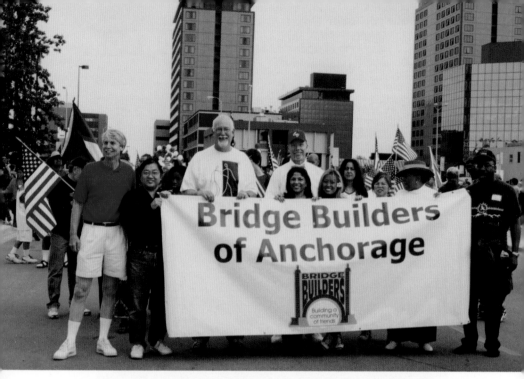

Preparing to lead the BridgeBuilders floats in Anchorage's annual July 4th parade. *From left*: Malcolm Roberts, in red shirt, longtime leader of BridgeBuilders; Paul Davis, BridgeBuilders cofounder, center in white shirt; and me.

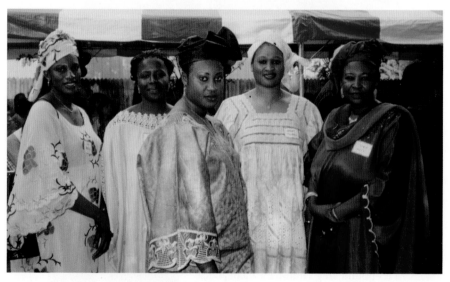

Anchorage's Gambian citizens

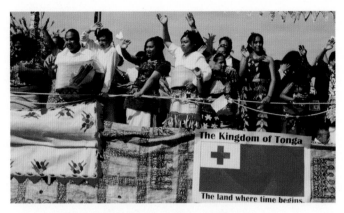

Anchorage's Tongan citizens

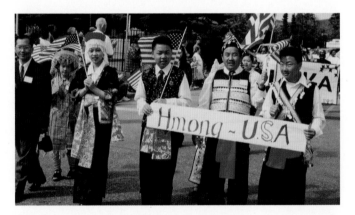

Anchorage's Hmong citizens

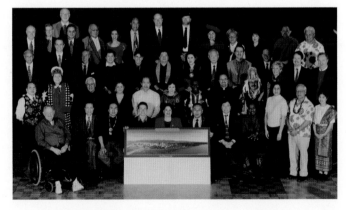

Anchorage leaders from more than two dozen
cultural groups celebrating the creation of
Anchorage's Pledge of Mutual Respect.

Today I will be healthy, happy, productive, growing, and giving.

—Rick Mystrom

My daily
morning
reminder
to myself.

Chapter 15

The Steps to a Healthy Life with Diabetes

Over the past 50 years, I've learned that living a healthy and happy life with diabetes involves five major steps. The *first step* is understanding diabetes. The *second step* is developing a positive attitude toward dealing with diabetes. The *third step* is beginning a healthy eating lifestyle—not a diet, just healthy eating habits you can live with the rest of your life. *The fourth step* is developing a healthy daily activity lifestyle—not necessarily becoming a runner or competitive athlete, but just moving a little more each day. The *fifth step* is starting a simple, structured, not necessarily strenuous, exercise lifestyle—one that's easy enough for you to do three to six days a week for 20 to 30 minutes.

I cover all these steps in detail in my companion book, *The New Diabetic Lifestyle* due out early 2014. That book focuses as much on Type 2 diabetes as on Type 1. Of special importance to Type 2 diabetics is the eating lifestyle to lower blood sugars and lose weight. The first two steps (*understanding diabetes* and a *positive attitude*) are so important I've included some parts of those two steps in both books.

Understanding Diabetes

What Happens When a Non-Diabetic Eats
(or Drinks) for Energy and Nourishment

The best way to understand diabetes is to first understand what happens when a *non-diabetic* eats food and converts it to energy. When a non-diabetic eats food, some of that food is converted to glucose and enters the bloodstream. When the glucose starts entering the bloodstream it triggers a rise in what is usually called blood sugar (also referred to as blood glucose).

In this book I use the two terms interchangeably. As the blood sugar begins to rise, the pancreas gets a signal to start producing insulin. Insulin is a hormone that allows the glucose that goes into the bloodstream to be absorbed through the walls of the bloodstream into the body's cells.

The pancreas obliges and produces insulin, which quickly gets into the bloodstream allowing the glucose (sugar) to get through the walls of the bloodstream into the cells to provide energy to the body and also to be stored as fat.

When sufficient insulin has been produced to allow the body to use the glucose in the bloodstream, and the level of glucose in the bloodstream drops back down to normal levels, the pancreas stops sending any more insulin to the bloodstream and the blood sugar stabilizes at that normal level. Normal is generally considered to be between 75 and 105 mg/dl (milligrams of glucose per deciliter of blood).

Think of it this way. It's like heating a house in the winter using a thermostat. When the house gets too cold the thermostat sends a message to the furnace that says "Turn on the heat." When the furnace brings the heat up to the set (or normal) temperature, the thermostat sends the signal to stop sending up heat.

That's the way things are supposed to work. But what if the pancreas doesn't produce any insulin or doesn't produce enough insulin? That's the challenge Type 1 or Type 2 diabetics have and borderline, or pre-diabetics will have if they don't take preventive action.

What Happens When a *Type 1* Diabetic Eats
(or Drinks) for Energy and Nourishment

What happens when an *untreated* Type 1 diabetic eats food is the same as for a non-diabetic—up to a point.

When a Type 1 diabetic eats food, some of that food is converted to glucose and absorbed into the blood stream just as it is with a non-diabetic. When the glucose starts entering the bloodstream it triggers a rise in blood sugar just as it does in a non-diabetic. As the blood sugar begins to rise, the pancreas gets a signal to start producing insulin so the body can use the energy the blood sugar will provide. This is where things change. The pancreas says, "Sorry, I don't do that anymore."

With no insulin being produced, the glucose can't get out of the blood-stream into the cells to provide energy to the body. Consequently, the blood sugar just gets higher and higher until eventually it reaches a level high enough (called the renal threshold) to spill into the kidneys and ultimately out the urethra as sugar in the urine. Thus, sugar in the urine is very often an early symptom that indicates diabetes. High blood sugars also trigger more frequent urination as the kidneys try to rid themselves of the excess sugar. A noticeable increase in the frequency of urination is often the first and most commonly noticed symptom of the onset of Type 1 diabetes.

Since the Type 1 diabetic in this example is not yet injecting insulin, the sugar continues to collect in the bloodstream but cannot get through the bloodstream walls to the body's cells, which need the energy and nour-ishment. The body's cells are screaming for nutrients so they can function. If the cells can't get the nourishment they now desperately need, the body starts burning its own fat. That doesn't work very well because fat molecules are very stable and hard to break down to function as energy supplies. In this process, they are often only partially broken down and the unused portions of the fat molecules are called ketones or acetones. When the ketones or acetones start showing up in the urine it indicates ketoacidosis, another result of untreated or poorly treated Type 1 diabetes. The undiag-nosed Type 1 diabetic then starts feeling lethargic, weak, and flu-like.

Prior to the discovery of insulin, the life expectancy of Type 1 diabetics was short indeed. Typically, they lived for just months and during that time they would be so weak and so sick that they couldn't perform routine life activities.

The discovery of insulin in the early 1920s by Doctors Frederick Banting and Charles Best, working at the University of Toronto, changed the life expectancy for Type 1 diabetics from just months to multiple decades and changed the quality and functionality of their lives dramatically.

It was in January, 1922 in Toronto, Canada that a 14-year-old boy, Leonard Thompson, was chosen as the first person with diabetes to receive insulin. The test was a dramatic success. Leonard, who before the insulin shots was near death, rapidly regained his strength and appetite. The team then expanded their testing to other volunteer diabetics, who reacted just as positively as Leonard to the insulin extract.

Magic stuff, that insulin. But one shot obviously doesn't solve the problem forever. A daily regimen of insulin injection or infusion will be required for Type 1 diabetics, hence the term *insulin-dependent*. As research continues and technology improves, this requirement for daily injections may change. But for now, your best path is to understand diabetes treatment as it is today. At this stage of medical advancement, most Type 1 diabetics will require outside insulin infusions or injections for the rest of their lives.

"The rest of one's life" always sounds intimidating but with the right attitude it can become a part of your life that will teach you so much about food that you can live healthier and longer than most of your peers. Because I've learned so much about food and health, I often tell people that I believe I'm healthier now than I would have been if I hadn't contracted Type 1 diabetes 50 years ago. It can be hard at first but this book will help your journey with diabetes be a good one.

What Happens When a *Type 2* Diabetic Eats
(or Drinks) for Energy and Nourishment

The process for a Type 2 diabetic before diagnosis and corrective action is also the same as for a non-diabetic—up to a point.

When an *untreated* Type 2 diabetic eats food, some of that food is absorbed into the bloodstream as glucose just as it does with a non-diabetic and a Type 1 diabetic. When the glucose starts entering the bloodstream it triggers a rise in blood sugar. As the blood sugar begins to rise, the pancreas gets a signal to start producing insulin. This is where things change. In a Type 2 diabetic the pancreas says, "I've been working too hard trying to produce all the insulin needed for all the glucose you've created. I'm worn out and I can't produce all the insulin you need. But I will produce what I can and hope it helps." Implicit in this message is that if the Type 2 diabetic will reduce the amount of glucose in the bloodstream, it will reduce the demand for insulin and the pancreas will likely be able to produce sufficient insulin to meet that demand.

This is essentially the difference between Type 1 diabetes and Type 2 diabetes. In a Type 1 diabetic, no insulin is produced. In a Type 2 diabetic the pancreas is producing some insulin but not enough to get *all* the glucose out of the bloodstream and into the cells that need the glucose for energy and nourishment.

This insufficiency of insulin may be related to weight, heredity, ethnicity, diet, sedentary lifestyle, or age. Most likely it's some combination of these characteristics. The most common characteristics of Type 2 diabetics are age and/or weight. Getting older and heavier is the most common journey to Type 2 diabetes. We can't do much about getting older; in fact, it's better than the alternative. But we can do something about the weight gain and that's a major focus of my companion book, *The New Diabetic Lifestyle*.

Characteristics of Type 2 Diabetes Compared to Type 1 Diabetes

Type 2 diabetes is typically much slower to develop than Type 1 and is therefore much more subtle. It may be present or developing for years before it is discovered. The blood sugars of a Type 2 diabetic don't typically (but may) get as high as the blood sugars of a Type 1 diabetic because the pancreas is producing some insulin. That means some of the sugar (glucose) in the blood is getting out of the bloodstream into the cells so the blood sugar readings of a Type 2 diabetic may be not nearly as high as the blood sugar readings of an uncontrolled Type 1 diabetic would be. In Type 2, the cells are also getting some energy from the bloodstream so an undiagnosed Type 2 diabetic may not feel as energy deprived as an undiagnosed Type 1.

Type 2 diabetics can sometimes be treated with oral medications that stimulate the pancreas to produce more insulin or make the insulin it is producing more effective. However, some Type 2 diabetics need insulin injections to supplement the insulin their bodies are producing. Whether a Type 2 diabetic is taking oral medications or injecting insulin, that diabetic will not have the big swings in blood sugar a Type 1 will have. That's because the partially working pancreas is a moderating force that makes the blood sugar of a Type 2 diabetic much more stable than that of a Type 1 but higher than that of a non-diabetic.

The best news of all for a Type 2 is that many, if not most, can eliminate all the symptoms of diabetes and rid themselves of the need of taking any medication by changing their lifestyle. Some may call that a cure of diabetes and some may say that's just eliminating the symptoms. Whichever is correct, the end result is that your body will act just like a healthy non-diabetic's and that's very good news.

Type 2 diabetes is usually contracted later in life than Type 1. Type 1 diabetics are typically diagnosed between birth and their late 20s and the onset is not usually related to lifestyle habits or weight. Type 2 diabetics are typically diagnosed from their 40s through the 70s and the onset is very often (but not always) related to a less-than-healthy lifestyle. When a Type 2 diabetic is diagnosed at a later age, his or her body is not as resilient as a person's who is diagnosed with Type 1 as a 20-year-old. This combination of factors means that Type 2 diabetics often have a smaller window of time than Type 1 diabetics to accept the diagnosis and create the new lifestyle necessary for a long, healthy life. (Later in this chapter I go into more detail on this issue.)

Are Type 2 Diabetics Who Use Insulin Really "Insulin-Dependent" or Are They Just "Insulin-Assisted"?

In the early stages of medical distinction between the two types of diabetes, I wish the term used to describe Type 2 diabetics who use insulin had been established as *insulin-assisted*, not *insulin-dependent*. As a Type 2 diabetic you may need that insulin assistance now but for many of you, if you can make some key changes in your eating lifestyle, you won't always need assistance from either insulin or oral medication.

In my companion book, *The New Diabetic Lifestyle*, I cover the five elements of a healthy life with diabetes. I get into detail on how to control blood sugar and live healthy with Type 1 diabetes. For Type 2 diabetics, I detail how to lose weight, lower blood sugar, and quite possibly lose all the symptoms of diabetes.

To assure your long-term good health as a Type 1 or Type 2 diabetic, you not only need to have an understanding of diabetes, but you also need to have a positive attitude about dealing with diabetes, whether Type 1 or Type 2.

A Positive Attitude, Your Best Prescription for a Healthy, Happy Life with Diabetes

Diabetes Shouldn't Dominate Your Life

It was April, 2004, about 40 years after my diagnosis as a diabetic. My family and I were in a small, beachfront restaurant in Lahaina on the island of Maui in Hawaii. My wife, Mary, and I had been married 34 years. Our oldest son, Nick, was 33, our son Rich was 30, and our daughter, Jen, was 27. Our family, including our soon-to-be son-in-law, Andy Scott, was on our almost annual vacation to Hawaii. We were eating lunch and I can't quite conjure up the reason for the comment, but my daughter, Jen, said, "Dad, you've never complained or made a big deal about having diabetes and that's made such a difference in our family life." My son Rich chipped in, "We all feel that way, Dad." Nick and Mary nodded in agreement and Andy, though he'd known me for less than a year, wisely weighed in on the positive side to atone for a minor problem we'd had the night before.

The significance of that comment was that even though I had had diabetes for more than 40 years, it was the first time I remember anyone really verbalizing the fact that I never complained about it.

My family had always been very supportive and helpful and I thought intuitively that they all felt I handled diabetes well. But the fact that it had never been verbalized was a testament to the fact that it was not a front-and-center issue in our family life. It was there but in the background. Mary and the kids were very much aware of the immediate dangers of extreme low blood sugar and of the more subtle symptoms of moderately low blood sugar. If I seemed a little disjointed in my conversation or a little irritable—both of which are, by the way, symptoms of low blood sugar—the kids would ask if my blood sugar was low.

I wondered sometimes if it had been smart of me to tell the kids that low blood sugar made me irritable because that became the question they often asked when they thought I was being unfairly mad at them. "Dad, is your blood sugar low?" It made me stop and think that maybe my little irritation wasn't caused by them.

The Mothers' Club and Their Secret to Long Lives

During my first term as mayor of Anchorage, Mary was invited to have tea one afternoon with a small group of ladies in Anchorage who called themselves "the Mothers' Club," though they were all grandmothers and many were great-grandmothers. Mary guessed that their average age was probably in the high 80s with a few in their low to mid 90s.

That night at dinner as Mary and I were talking, I asked her about her tea with the Mothers' Club. She said she'd had a delightful time. The ladies were to a person pleasant, positive, and friendly and all were very alert. She also reported that they all loved living in Anchorage and they thought that I was doing a great job as mayor. Not only that, but they thought that the mayor before me and the mayor before that had also done great jobs. In fact, they were pretty sure that every mayor in Anchorage's history had done a great job.

After they finished reminiscing and glowing about Anchorage, their children, their grandchildren, and life in general, Mary asked them the perfect question: "What do you attribute your long lives and good health to?" The answer surprised her. They all agreed that it was a positive attitude. That clearly explained why they thought every mayor in Anchorage's history had done a great job.

They all pretty much agreed that they weren't complainers, worriers, or critics. Rather, they saw themselves as being supportive, encouraging, and caring. They felt better because they made others feel better. That was their prescription for a long, happy life.

Passing along a Positive Attitude

Every day in our lives, each of us has the opportunity to make others feel better. Whether it's a server in a restaurant, a clerk in a retail store, or just someone you're passing on the sidewalk. A kind word, a compliment, or even just a smile that makes them feel better will make you feel better too—guaranteed. I've found that it's a lot easier to have a positive attitude about diabetes if you have a positive attitude about life and pass that attitude on to others.

"Spread the Love—Keep the Change" — *Nick Mystrom, 2002*

About 35 years ago, Mary and I and our kids were having dinner at a small restaurant near the Anchorage airport. It was a Sunday afternoon. We had just come from swimming at a local pool. We had all showered and everybody looked fresh and neat. The kids were well-behaved. As I looked around the restaurant, I saw that only one other person, an older man, was eating there. Looking at the menu, I realized the dinner for the five of us was going to be over $20. This was going to be a bit of a stretch for us because our budget when our family ate out was $10 for all of us. We could usually accomplish that by sharing meals and diluting the kid's lemonades or making our own lemonade with free lemon slices and sugar.

This food we had ordered was way above our budget. But I never did know how much it cost because when I asked for the check, the waitress told me that the other gentleman in the restaurant had paid for our meal. She told us that he had remarked about how neat and well-behaved the kids were and what a nice family we seemed to be. Then she told us that he was the owner and was from out of town. It was especially meaningful to me because we were the only paying customers in the restaurant. I never was able to thank him but I've never forgotten that little gesture.

As our kids have grown, I've reminded them of that event a number of times. As they've grown into independent adults, they each go out of their way to help others while asking for nothing in return.

In fact, this small kindness had such an impact on our oldest son, Nick, that when he was in his early 30s he started an organization called the Karma Club. It's dedicated to doing something good for people as you see a need or opportunity and asking nothing more than that the recipient of the kindness pass on a kindness to someone else. Their motto is "Spread the Love. Keep the Change." Nick's organization has helped many people around the country with some small and some very big kindnesses and many are described on the website karmaclub.org.

It all started with one person buying one meal for one family. Every small gesture you make to another person has the potential to be passed on many times over, making the world, and you in it, just a little bit better. As a diabetic, you'll find that you'll have many opportunities to share your positive experiences with others. In doing so you can add to the quality of their lives and you'll find that with each of those moments of sharing your life gets better too.

On the opening page of the Karma Club website, Nick refers to that small kindness in the restaurant 35 years ago. Here's his memory of it.

> When I was around eight, my family and I were eating at a restaurant in Anchorage. At the time, we were very tight on money, and my father's budget for all five of us was 10 dollars. I can remember making lemonade with the water the waitress brought us by using sugar packets and lemons so none of us had to buy beverages. When it came time to pay the bill, the waitress said it was already paid by the only other person in the restaurant, the owner. He had told the waitress what a nice family we were and had bought our dinner.

> That was years ago, and to this day, my father still talks about that dinner a stranger bought for us at an Anchorage restaurant. About five years ago, Dad asked all us kids to stop buying him Christmas and birthday presents and to just buy a meal for a family in honor of the man who bought us a meal and, without knowing, planted the seed for the Karma Club.

> Every single day, I encounter someone in need. Maybe they need their driveway shoveled or their teeth fixed, maybe they need some help when their car breaks down or a plane ticket to see their ailing

mother, maybe they don't quite have enough for the groceries or maybe, just maybe, there's a father eating with his family at a restaurant in Anchorage, Alaska and staring nervously at a dinner bill. The purpose of the Karma Club is to get people to see these situations as opportunities to do the right thing and help someone out just for the sake of helping them out.

The Karma Club is founded in honor of my father and in honor of that man who bought our dinner 25 years ago and changed my outlook and perspective in doing so.

—Nick Mystrom

As you're dealing with the challenges of making your life healthier with diabetes, you'll be happier if diabetes isn't your total focus. Every chance you get, try to do some little, thoughtful deed for someone else. Each time you do, it will help put you in touch with your worth in life. And some of those little helpful deeds will always be remembered by the recipients and may then be passed forward to someone else.

It's easier to be positive about diabetes if you're also aware of trying to make your life better in other areas. My reminder to myself each morning in the shower is this simple statement: *"Today I'm going to be healthy, happy, productive, growing, and giving."* This reminds me every morning that I have to do what I can to maintain my health as a diabetic but it also reminds me that my life is full and diabetes is just one element.

The Special Importance of Attitude for Older Type 2 Diabetics

Type 2 diabetes is typically considered less serious than Type 1. The reasons are, on the surface, quite obvious. With Type 1 diabetes no insulin is produced and insulin injections or infusions are essential to survival. With Type 2 diabetes some insulin is produced by the pancreas. Oral medications can often normalize blood sugars by stimulating the production of more insulin. Not only can oral medications be effective with Type 2, but oftentimes, a change in eating habits, loss of weight, and more physical activity can normalize blood sugar levels and preclude the need for either oral medication or insulin injections.

Most Type 2 diabetics I talk to have a strong aversion to starting insulin injections. That's very natural. But at some point in time if improvements in eating habits, increases in physical activity, or taking oral medication all fail to normalize blood sugars, some method of insulin injection or infusion is not only necessary but also desirable. Most Type 2 diabetics who reach that point do settle into an injection routine that, after a short period of time, becomes comfortable and not too burdensome. They also tell me that they feel better, have more energy, and sleep better.

I believe that considering Type 2 diabetes less serious than Type 1 is a danger that very often leads to significant health problems and a shorter life for those Type 2 diabetics who don't very quickly develop an understanding and a positive approach to dealing with their challenge.

So why is Type 2 so serious and why is a positive attitude of special importance to older Type 2 diabetics? To start with, Type 2 diabetes usually develops in people over 40 years old and is much more common in people who are overweight. When Type 2 diabetes manifests itself in older people, it's usually a result of long-developing, at least moderately unhealthy eating habits, and a slowly diminishing level of activity.

In my personal observations and discussions, a significant number of older male Type 2 diabetics were active in athletics in their youth. With that high level of activity, they had the luxury of eating whatever they wanted, whenever they wanted, and as much as they wanted without the resulting weight gain that non-athletes would have experienced. But after the competitive activity in their lives stopped, their eating portions often did not.

Two major issues are at play here: (1) Long-term bad habits are hard to break and, (2) when you get diabetes at a later age, your body is not as healthy and resilient as the body of someone who may get diabetes much earlier in life.

If you're an older Type 2 diabetic and you have habits to break, you must realize that you have a smaller window of time than a younger diabetic would have to change those habits. You can't take five or 10 years to change your habits and normalize your blood sugars.

Contrast that small window of time for a Type 2 diabetic with my personal experience having contracted Type 1 Diabetes at age 20. When I first got diabetes, I tried to learn everything I could about what I should do, but self-testing wasn't available so I never knew what my blood sugars were except for once or twice a year when I visited a doctor and had a lab test for blood sugar done. And quite frankly they were often in the 200-to-300 mg/dl range. But because I was young, active, and healthy, I had quite a few years to learn how to control my blood sugars without much damage apparently done.

I have mentioned that the one problem I have as a result of having diabetes for 50 years is a diminished sensitivity in my feet called neuropathy. My podiatrist tells me that he feels that may be because of my high blood sugars at an early age. So although a younger person has a larger window of time to adapt, it shouldn't be interpreted as a total free ride.

I don't mean to imply that a young Type 1 diabetic should take a long time to adapt to having diabetes. With the current technology you can deal well with diabetes a lot faster than I did nearly 50 years ago. But if it does take some time for young Type 1 diabetics to accept and adapt, it will harm them less than older Type 2 diabetics who take the same length of time to adapt. I know a half dozen people in Anchorage who contracted Type 2 diabetes in their 50s or early 60s and died within 10 to 12 years. That should not happen. Being diagnosed as a Type 2 diabetic at any age can be your ticket to a longer, healthy life—not a sentence to a shorter, unhealthy life. It's up to you. It's a wake-up call that says start now—don't wait.

A positive attitude and a willingness to learn and act on what you learn can be your ticket to eliminating the symptoms of Type 2 diabetes or to living a long, happy life with Type 2 diabetes.

Some Promises You Should Consider

Diabetes doesn't have to be a hindrance or a barrier to you or your family's activities. You can actually live a healthier and more active life than non-diabetics because by measuring your blood sugar you'll start learning how each type of food you eat impacts your body.

Living a healthy, active life with diabetes starts with you. It starts with a promise. Here are some thoughts to consider as you decide what promise works for you.

1. I accept the fact that I have diabetes. I know that I have to be a little smarter and a little more careful about what I eat than other people. I also know that if I test my blood appropriately, I will know more about what foods will keep me healthy than non-diabetics will know. I will understand the impact of foods and exercise on my health and my weight.

2. I will develop good exercise and eating patterns that I will eventually turn into habits that I can maintain. I recognize that neither my exercise nor my eating patterns will be perfect, but I know they don't have to be. They just have to be good.

3. I promise that I will not complain about having diabetes but that I will learn from it and if I apply what I learned, I know that I will feel better, be healthier, and be trimmer than most non-diabetics.

4. I promise that I will not let diabetes keep me from doing anything in the world that I want to do with my life. I know that if I keep this promise I can live a healthy, active, and fulfilling life with diabetes.

That's a lot to think about but keep referring back to this chapter. If you can make and keep your own promise from these ideas, every day will dawn brighter.

As I've spoken to groups about diabetes and mentioned my promise never to complain about being a diabetic, it has become the single point that doctors in the audience have most often commented positively about. Their typical reaction is, "If I could get all my patients to think that way, they would be so much healthier." Attitude is more important than perfection in eating habits. Attitude is more important than absolute dedication to exercise. If you can have or can develop a good attitude about your diabetes and your life, you will live healthy, live well, and live long with diabetes.

The Other Three Steps to a Healthy Lifestyle with Diabetes

The five steps to a healthy, happy life with diabetes that have been so helpful to me, will, I hope, be equally helpful to you. The first two steps, an understanding of diabetes and a positive attitude, I've touched on in this book. The next three steps, 3, 4, and 5, are matters of lifestyle. *Step 3* is a healthy eating lifestyle—not a diet, just healthy eating habits you can live with the rest of your life. *Step 4* is a healthy daily activity lifestyle—not necessarily becoming a runner or competitive athlete, but just moving a little more each day. *Step 5* is starting a simple, structured, nonstrenuous exercise lifestyle. My companion book, *The New Diabetic Lifestyle*, provides detailed information on all five steps and will tell you what to eat and how to eat. It also covers simple steps for creating a more active lifestyle. And finally, it provides a simple, not-too-hard exercise program designed for older Type 2 diabetics who may never have had a structured exercise program or may never even have been in a gym.

I'm writing *The New Diabetic Lifestyle* to share what I've learned about foods and healthy living from 50 years and 60,000 blood tests as a Type 1 diabetic. But what I've learned has turned out to be every bit as important for Type 2 diabetics who want to lose weight and lower blood sugars. Not only will *The New Diabetic Lifestyle* be very informative for Type 1 diabetics who want to better control their blood sugars and live a long, healthy life, but it will also be life-changing for Type 2 diabetics who want to lower their blood sugars, lose weight, and live healthier.

A song is no song 'til you sing it,
A bell is no bell 'til you ring it;
And the love in your heart,
Wasn't put there to stay;
For love isn't love 'til you
Give it away.

—Oscar Hammerstein

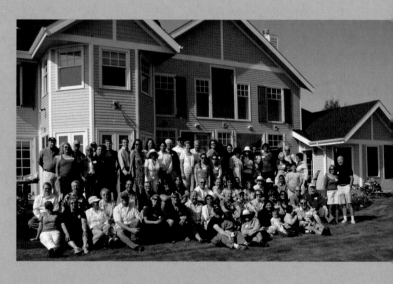

My Anchorage East Rotary Club and their families at our 2011 "Day at the Lake." At our lake house in the Matunuska Valley.

Summary

I wrote this book in hopes of inspiring and empowering diabetics to be healthy, happy, productive, growing, and giving. I hope I've been successful in helping you in some modest way.

At the start of this chapter I communicated my daily reminders to myself right under the chapter name. These reminders, I believe, have been great contributors to my health, happiness, and fulfillment. They also provide a good summary of the philosophical approach I have attempted to convey in this book.

I'd like to leave you with an explanation of these reminders in hopes that you will consider choosing some variation of these for yourself. The five reminders for me are to strive every day to be "healthy, happy, productive, growing, and giving."

Healthy

I don't think I need additional explanation about the importance of striving for health since the biggest part of both this book and *The New Diabetic Lifestyle* focuses heavily on being healthy.

Happy

What I've learned about happiness over the past 40 years is that I shouldn't just pursue happiness. Happiness is not a goal. It's a result. If I pursue and achieve the other four reminders, happiness presents itself to me. In other words, if I continue to try to be as healthy as I can, if I feel I am productive, if I am growing mentally and emotionally, and if I focus on giving, happiness is the result.

Productive

If I feel each day I'm adding something to the human experience, If I feel I'm accomplishing my "to do" list, if I feel I completed what I set out to do that day, then I end the day feeling productive. That feeling makes my evenings better. It makes my vacations better, and as I mentioned earlier, it adds to my happiness.

Growing

Growing to me means developing a deeper understanding of life. It means learning from experiences, from travel, from books, from news media, from taking risks, but most of all from conversations with others. It took me decades—too long—to learn that the key to good, learning, fulfilling conversations was not just being an interesting talker but more important was being an interested listener. It was my wife, Mary, who brought that to my front-of-mind awareness when she described a friend as being both interesting and interested. Being able to feel each day that I'm growing adds noticeably to my happiness.

Giving

Of my five reminders, giving is the most important to me and it's appropriate that I end this memoir with it. I find it very hard to say no to people or organizations who ask me to help them. In the smaller picture of my life, this has been a little frustrating for me but now as I approach 70 and observe through a more distant lens, I realize how much meaning and purpose saying yes has given me. In fact, in a lot of ways it's defined my life. To a great degree, I credit Rotary for continually reminding me of the importance of giving and of service to others. I've been a member of Anchorage East Rotary Club for nearly 40 years now and my life, and I know millions of others' lives, are better because of Rotary.

No one has described the importance of giving better than Oscar Hammerstein, a creator, along with Richard Rodgers, of a number of great American musicals. I read his thought on giving over 50 years ago and it still works its way to the front of my mind every few years. That thought appears at the start of this summary chapter.

I am of the opinion that my life belongs to the whole community, and that as long as I live it is it is my privilege to do for it whatever I can ... for the harder I work, the more I live. I rejoice in life for its own sake. Life is no brief candle for me. It is a sort of splendid torch which I have got a hold of for the moment, which I want to make burn brightly as possible before turning it over to future generations."

—George Bernard Shaw

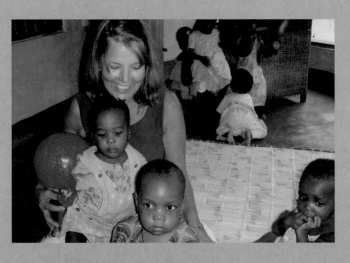

My wife, Mary, caring for young, orphaned, children at the Malawi Children's Village, founded by Tom and Ruth Nighswander of Anchorage and supported largely by Alaskans. Many of the pre-school age children have malaria or are HIV positive.

Epilogue

My post-mayor years have continued to follow the patterns of my past. Lots of fun physical activity, community involvement, and a moderate gym workout three to six times a week keep me healthy, fit, and emotionally fulfilled. But above all of that is the joy of being active and involved with our growing extended family.

Every summer we have reunions at our lake house with some or all of our family. Being an active participant in all the water sports with our kids, our grandkids, our nephews and nieces is a true blessing.

My good health and physical condition as well as Mary's good physical condition also allow us to take part in sports and activities year-round. I'm enjoying golf more than ever and love the two or three golf trips a year I take with friends. Mary and I are improving our waterskiing and wake surfing in the summer and our cross-country skiing and ice skating in the winter. We also love downhill skiing in Colorado and Alaska and both smile when we talk about the free skiing we'll get at many resorts when we turn 80.

We've hiked the Grand Canyon from the rim down to the Colorado River, stayed overnight at Phantom Ranch, and hiked back up the next day—something every American should do if possible. We also took a trip around America in our SUV with our bikes hung on the back. We took guided bike trips around Nantucket and Martha's Vineyard. And as we circled our spectacular country and approached a small town that looked appealing, we'd park the SUV on the outskirts and ride our bikes into the town for a meal or just some sightseeing.

Certainly the most exciting and fulfilling trip Mary and I have taken since the last of my terms ended was a four-week experience in the small country of Malawi in Africa in January 2007. We went with the president of Alaska Pacific University, Doug North, his wife, Ellen Cole, and nine university students. The purpose of the trip was to volunteer at the Malawi Children's Village, an orphanage and school started by Dr. Tom and Ruth Nighswander of Anchorage.

The children of Malawi had borne the suffering in the years previous to our visit from the devastation of a drought which decimated their maize crop, the core food of their existence. That crop failure combined with the deaths of many young fathers from AIDS and the continual scourge of malaria left many of the country's children without parents or with just a mother who couldn't feed or care for them. Malawi Children's Village provides care, food, and education through what Americans would call the high school level. To help the preschool age kids at the orphanage and teach the school-age kids was a uniquely fulfilling experience for both Mary and me.

In Malawi we met an Afghani family, a father, mother, and four smart, beautiful daughters. The father (I'm going to avoid using first or last names in this book to protect their identities) had been a teacher at a girls school in Afghanistan founded by a former Alaska Pacific University student, Nate York. In Afghanistan, giving girls an opportunity to learn is a very threatening prospect to the Taliban and the mullahs.

One day, shortly before we met them in Malawi, the father was visited by town leaders. He was told that he must sell his daughters to these town leaders or he and his wife would be killed and they would take their daughters. The next night the family took provisions needed for a few days and escaped Afghanistan on foot. With Nate's help they were able to get to Malawi without a visa and start school at the Alaska Children's Village.

A very caring and generous woman, whose name I don't know, took their education as her responsibility and paid for the girls to attend a high-quality—and very expensive— international school in Blantyre, the largest city in Malawi. The family's story is still evolving but the prospects for a happy ending are improving. Someday they may be able to work their way through the discouraging labyrinth of our American immigration process.

It was there, in Malawi, I experienced one of only two negative experiences with Medtronic in the 30 years I have been their customer. My insulin pump just went blank the second day we were there. Maybe it was the stifling heat-humidity combination. It was never below the mid eighties Fahrenheit and not much below 95 percent relative humidity. Sleeping in a hut under a mosquito net gave no relief. I called Medtronic via a satellite phone on January 7. The customer service representative gave me a protocol for restarting it but that failed. I called the rep back later that day. He said they would send me a replacement pump. Great. I gave them a post office box number in a small nearby town.

Three days later I called to see if it was on the way. It wasn't. The rep said the international division had e-mailed him and said they couldn't ship it because it was a P.O. box and not an address. I then described in detail what my location was and told the representative that I had only a five-day supply of syringes. I had brought a packet of ten syringes with me in case of a pump problem.

The next day, Tuesday in Malawi, Monday in the United States, I tried to call the international division of Medtronic. They were closed: Martin Luther King Day. I called again the next day. I was getting very frustrated. Each phone call was 20 or more minutes with no discernable progress. I called again the following day. Couldn't get through to the guy I'd been talking to. The rep I did reach said we needed to start over. Five days now. Nothing was even off the ground. The only thing that had happened so far was some e-mails between the international division and the domestic division.

The next morning I made my sixth call to try to make something happen. I got hold of a supervisor, Rob Castro. He was a miracle worker. He worked way past his shift to develop a strategy and woke up early the next morning and followed up from home. Whatever he did worked. Two days later a junked-up pickup, steam coming out of its overheated engine, bumped along the pothole-filled muddy road and approached our hut. A skinny

Malawaian man with a big smile hopped out and ran toward me. He said he was told to get this package to me fast. It was, of course, a new insulin pump. Thank you, Rob.

My life continues with adventure and fulfillment. As a person facing grim health predictions 50 years ago, I've been truly blessed. In fact, I'm convinced now that I would not be as healthy or as fit as I am had I not contracted diabetes. I've had some doctors react with skepticism when I've said that. But I sincerely believe it's true. My hope is that this book as well as my companion book *The New Diabetic Lifestyle* will give other diabetics a clear path to be able to make that same statement about their health 30, 40, or 50 years from now.

The Enjoyment of
a Healthy Lifestyle

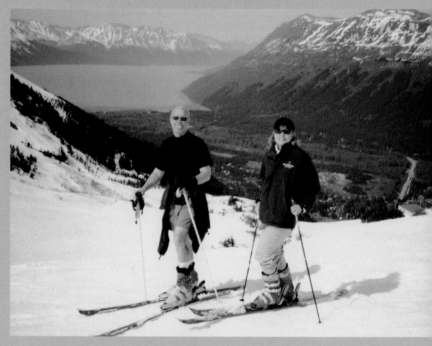

Mary and I spring skiing at Alyeska,
Alaska's biggest ski area.

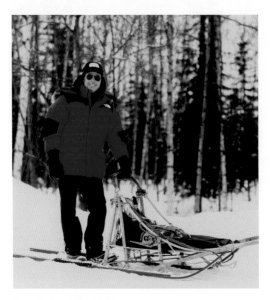

Ready for a short dog-mushing run, one of my
favorite winter activities

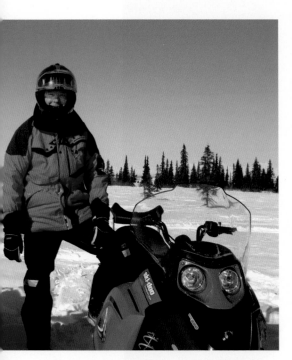

Taking a break from snowmobiling with
friends near Talkeetna, Alaska

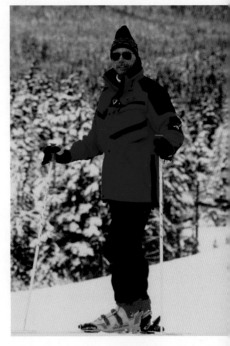

Mid-winter skiing at Alyeska

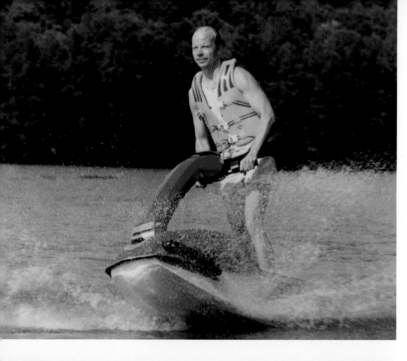

Jet skiing on Lake Hamilton near Hot Springs, Arkansas. I can very conveniently and harmlessly disconnect my insulin pump for a couple of hours for activities like this.

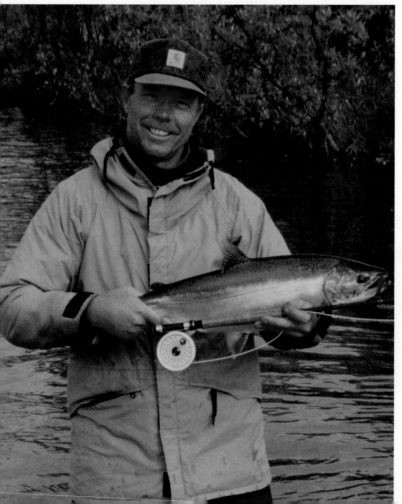

One of many nice silver salmon caught on a week-long float trip on the Kanektok River in Western Alaska.

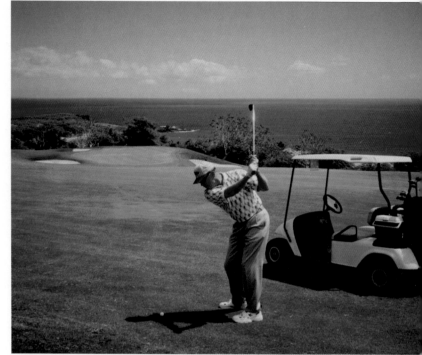

Golfing in Hawaii on an annual trip with a dozen or so close Alaskan friends.

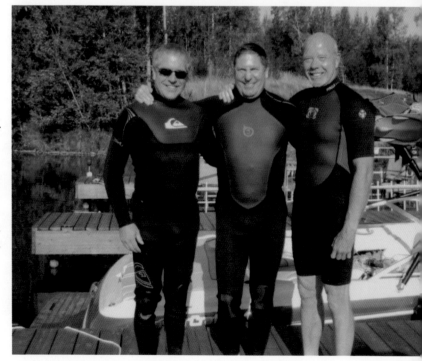

Ready for an afternoon of water-skiing, wake boarding, and wake surfing with my close friends, Dave Young and Rick Pollock

The Family
Rewards of a
Healthy Lifestyle

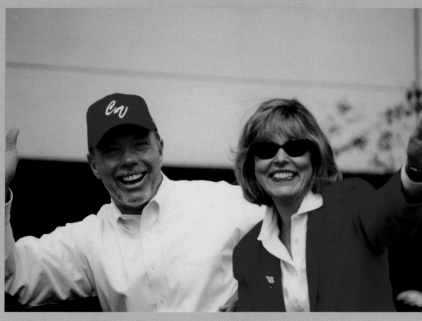

Mary and I in Anchorage's July 4th parade just
after finishing my last term as Mayor.

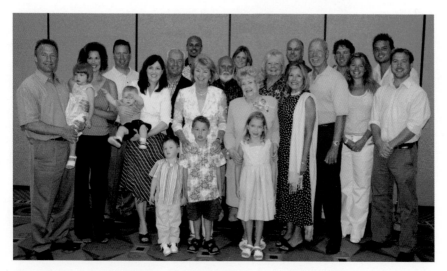

Our family at my mom's 90th birthday party

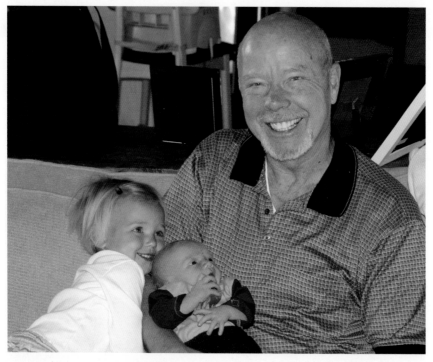

The joy of being a grandpa. With Lily and Boden, our first two grandkids.

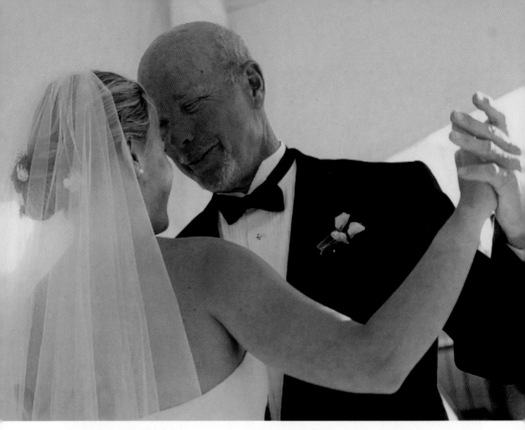

Dancing with my daughter, Jen, on her wedding day.

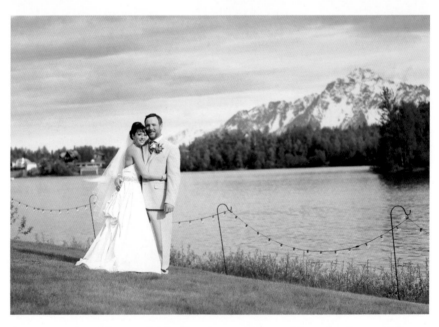

Our son, Rich and his new bride, Kari, in our front yard just after their wedding.

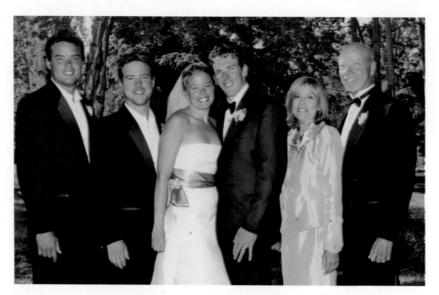

Our daughter, Jen and her new husband, Andy Scott with Mary and I and our two sons, Nick and Rich.

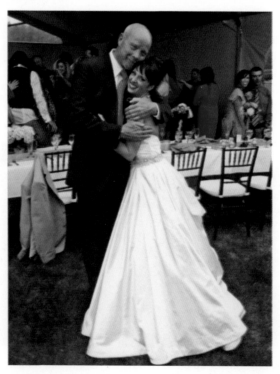

A precious hug with my new daughter-in-law, Kari.

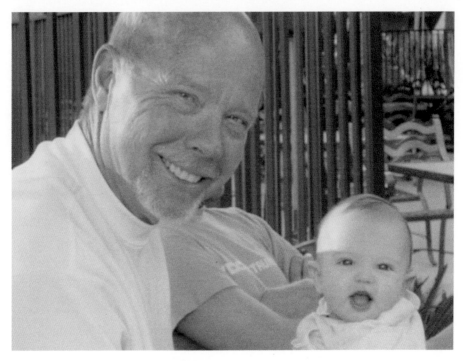

With Lily, our first granddaughter.

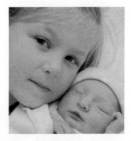

Our niece, Jayden Breaux with her little sister, Kenley, our newest family member.

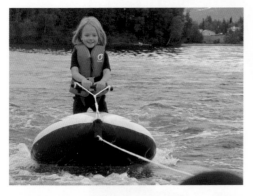

Granddaughter, Lily, getting up on water-ski trainer for the first time.

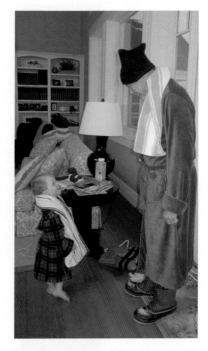

Grandson, Boden, and I getting ready to go out for a winter hot-tub dip.

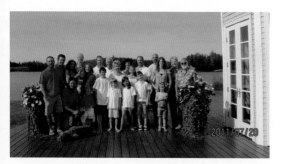

Our 2011 family reunion that was one of the great joys and rewards of my healthy life with diabetes.

Photo courtesy of Kathy Sage

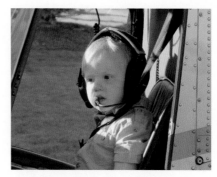

Our grandson, Boden. Ready for take-off from our front yard in the helicopter of good friends, Jerry Winchester and Dianne Louise.

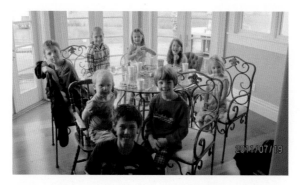

The newest generation of our extended family and even more motivation to stay healthy for the next 25 or more years.

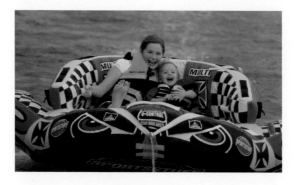

Niece, Brianna Lindemann and granddaughter, Lily Scott loving the ride.

Two of the many reasons we love living in Alaska

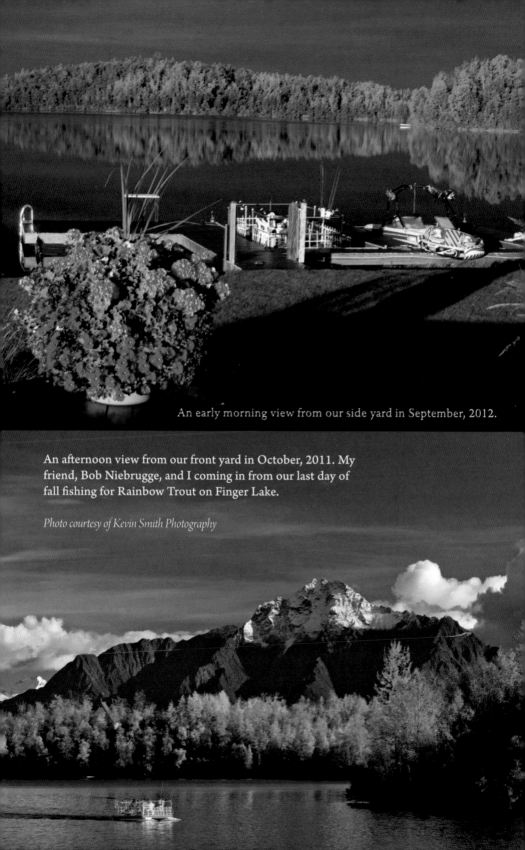

An early morning view from our side yard in September, 2012.

An afternoon view from our front yard in October, 2011. My friend, Bob Niebrugge, and I coming in from our last day of fall fishing for Rainbow Trout on Finger Lake.

Photo courtesy of Kevin Smith Photography

*I extend my gratitude to the thousands
of volunteers and supporters who have
so willingly embraced my projects
and dreams for Alaska and helped
give me the wonderful life that
I've been blessed with.*

—Rick Mystrom

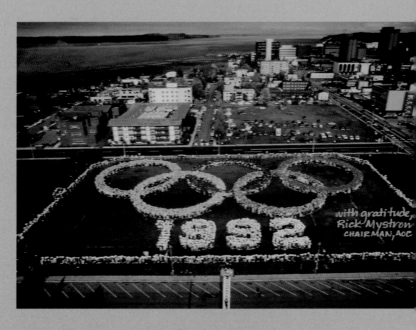

About 3,500 Anchorage citizens showed up at the Anchorage Park Strip on
a Sunday afternoon, September 21, 1986, to show their support of our
Olympic bid and become part of Anchorage's human Olympic rings.
It was extraordinarily successful and became the conclusion of
our presentation to the IOC.

Photo courtesy of Clark Mischler

Appendix

Bringing Honor to Anchorage
The New York Times, November 1986

Bud Greenspan, author of this personal and warmly enthusiastic report on the dramatic impact made by Alaskans last month during the 91st meeting of the International Olympic Committee in Lausanne, Switzerland, is a power in both the entertainment and sports worlds.

A movie producer and director of great acclaim, earlier this year he released his documentary film *16 Days for Glory*, which won acclaim for the moving way in which it captured the excitement and drama of the 1984 Olympic Summer Games in Los Angeles.

In Lausanne, Greenspan was able to see firsthand the zest and vigor of the Anchorage pursuit of the Winter Games. This report of his encounter with Alaskans in Switzerland is scheduled later this month for national publication and syndication.

Bid for Olympics mirrored courage of the pioneers

The New York Times, November 1986 By Bud Greenspan

One evening before you sit down to watch television and have nothing better to do, pour yourself some champagne or a stein of beer and raise your glass in a toast to a marvelous group of Alaskans who did America proud in Lausanne, Switzerland three weeks ago. There, this joyful contingent of more than 100 men and women from Anchorage, most of whom paid their own way, showed the high rollers and deal makers from six other cities bidding for the 1992 Winter Olympic Games what talent, pride and courage is all about. They brought tears to the eyes of those of us who on rare occasions think back to the noble pioneers who prevailed at Valley Forge and survived the awful trek over the desolate plains to California when America was young.

The Anchorage people are America's present-day pioneers. Some of them who came to Lausanne were Native-born Alaskans, but most of them originally came from Chicago, Indianapolis, Salt Lake City and countless other places in the Lower 48 to make a life for themselves in the new frontier. For a time during the oil boom in the 1970s Alaska was America's most prosperous state, but in recent years it has fallen on hard times. That is why there were so many raised eyebrows when the United States Olympic Committee selected Anchorage over Lake Placid, N.Y., Salt Lake City and Reno-Tahoe, Nev., as the United States representative to bid for the 1992 Winter Olympics against the likes of Albertville, France; Falun, Sweden; Cortina D'Ampezzo, Italy; Berchtesgaden, Germany; Sofia, Yugoslavia; and Lillehammer, Norway. Brilliantly clothed in their white fur-trimmed blue parkas and seemingly everywhere, the Anchorage people were the most visible and enthusiastic group in Lausanne. They knew their city was the "new kid on the block" and they smiled the good smile as Gina Lollobrigida was flown in to promote Cortina's bid and watched respectfully as Prime Minister Jacques Chirac of France joined triple gold medal winner Jean Claude Killy in telling the world press why Albertville should host the 1992 Winter Games. There were no front-page superstars from Anchorage, but their joy and vision brought more attention to their presentation than any other city's bid.

The Anchorage contingent knew all about the odds against a first-time candidate getting the nod from IOC members, but these are people who for the most part picked up stakes years ago to face odds in a new land that was far more formidable than competing against the likes of Gina Lollobrigida and Jean Claude Killy. Weighing even more heavily against Alaska's bid and receiving more than token recognition was the historic fact that Montreal and Los Angeles were the summer hosts in 1976 and 1984 and Lake Placid and Calgary the winter hosts in 1980 and 1988. Veteran Olympic watchers knew there was no way that North America would receive the Olympic bid five successive times within a 16-year period.

But for a city which had fewer than 2,000 people in 1920 and now boasts a population of 250,000, these obstacles had little meaning. The contingent's bid for the 1992 Games was a piece of cake compared to the odds that faced its members going to the Last Frontier. The beauty of the Anchorage people was their lovely combination of professionalism and naivete. Overcoming insurmountable odds is part of the drill when you become a pioneer. The main credo when you enter the pioneer arena is that age-old axiom, "Some men see things as they are and ask 'Why?' Others dream things that never were and ask, 'Why not?'" So the Alaskans asked, "Why not?" The people from Anchorage showed they were for real earlier this year in a preliminary IOC session in Seoul, South Korea, when a large group of Alaskans paid their own way in a dramatic show of support for the city's candidacy. They knocked the IOC members on their ears with their daring presentation which included the delightful antics of a tap-dancing moose, the city's mascot.

However, besides the glamorous blue parkas and dancing moose, Anchorage had solid technical credentials to host the games. Its winter sports facilities are top drawer and second to no city on this earth. Furthermore, the Olympic games are more than facilities, transportation, housing, athletes and foreign spectators. The Olympic games are people and not one of the candidates wanted the games more than Anchorage and especially all of the Alaskan people.

What other bidding city could offer an untouched, beautiful wilderness just a half-hour's drive from the Olympic sites with centuries-old glaciers creating a fantasy world within sight of magnificent Mount McKinley, the tallest mountain in North America? When the Candidacy Committee of Anchorage led by its chairman Rick Mystrom, the head of the largest advertising agency in Alaska, finished its presentation in Lausanne, its members were sure they had overcome the overwhelming obstacles that confronted them. Several IOC members promised their votes. Almost all of the Anchorage contingent ran to the telexes and telephones to send the word back home, certain they were going to pull the biggest upset in Olympic history. For the next two days they lobbied without really knowing how to lobby — just sheer joyful exuberance that was contagious. They did not know or believe that those same IOC members who promised votes were speaking from the emotion of the moment and would later reflect that their "real world" commitments were elsewhere.

Bidding for the Olympic games is not only big business but the results are usually safe and traditional. One is more likely to believe the rumors that if Paris were not awarded the Summer Olympics, the IOC members would appease the French by selecting Albertville as the winter site, or that the East European block would change its vote after a token first-round pledge to Sofia and later vote for Paris in exchange for a 1994 Winter Games vote for Leningrad. Every day in Lausanne there were talks of new front runners and rumors of deals, but the Anchorage people remained enthusiastic, certain that right wins over might. Two nights before the voting, the Alaskans held a dinner to honor their candidacy committee and supporters. Before the dinner there was a cocktail party that was more like a victory rally before a Notre Dame football game. Each speaker was cheered to the rafters and the momentum of their fervor was intoxicating and, for a time, even I began to think that perhaps there might be justice in the world and God would smile down on this happy band of Alaskans. But when the speechmaking and singing was over and this joyful group of pioneers went to dinner, a deep sense of sadness came over me. For these good people, who more than any other contingent fulfilled the Olympic philosophy of entering the arena, making the attempt and pursuing excellence, had not the slightest sense that in less than 40 hours their bubble would burst and they would be eliminated from contention after only two rounds.

So I asked Rick Mystrom to invite his contingent to a screening of "16 Days of Glory," our film on the 1984 Los Angeles Olympic Games, that was scheduled to be shown the next morning for the world press, just a few hours before the announcement of the winning Olympic cities. I thought this would be my contribution to their effort … to have two hours of watching the grandeur and glory of the greatest of athletic events and to perhaps reflect, win or lose, on the nobility of what they had done and what they must continue to do. When the film was over, many (with tears in their eyes) came over to me, laughing and crying, and for a brief moment were sober in their thoughts. My last words to them were those that sent the ancient Greeks into the Olympic arena so many years ago: "Ask not alone for victory, ask for courage, for if you endure you bring honor to yourself, even more you bring honor to us all." At that point I believe many of them for the first time realized that perhaps their time was not 1992 but 1994.

After the voting was over, one reporter came over to Rick Mystrom and asked what he and his Alaskans were going to do. Speaking for all of them, he replied, "We'll get back home on Sunday, take Monday off and on Tuesday start working for 1994." So one night when you've got nothing better to do, raise your glass in a toast to that happy band of Americans from Anchorage, those pioneers who entered the arena, dreamed a dream and fought the good fight. For one week in Lausanne they showed the world what American pioneers were like those many years ago … and because of it they brought honor to us all.

Index